Dance

To

Live

Book cover photos:

Shelly S. Harrington – professional dance instructor in Largo, Florida.

John P. Lenhart M.D.

Cover design:

Paula Keyser – keyserproductions.com

Dance like no one is watching

Dance

David J. Lenhart (signature)

To

Live

John P. Lenhart, M.D.

Copyright © 2007 by John P. Lenhart, M.D.

| ISBN # | Softcover | 1-930822-31-6 |
| ISBN13 # | Softcover | 978-1-930822-31-3 |

This book was printed in the United States of America

To order additional copies of this book, contact:
Medfo Publishing, a division of Medfo Inc.
6110 9th st N
St Petersburg, Florida 33703

1-800-332-7400
www.antiagingrevolution.com

CONTENTS

ACKNOWLEDGEMENT

I would like to thank my editor, Diane Marcou, for her help in smoothing out my sentences. Diane helped make this book easier to read and I appreciate her professionalism greatly.

DISCLAIMER

This book is not intended to act as a substitute for advice from your personal physician. The information presented in this book is for educational purposes only and not intended to diagnose or treat disease, or to render medical advice. Before starting any exercise or anti-aging program please consult your personal physician to determine the appropriateness of the program based upon your personal medical history.

FOREWORD

Everyone agrees that when you are enjoying yourself in what you are doing, you are truly living. I believe that dancing is a way to achieve that enjoyment and at the same time, glean the rewards of good health. This book is about dancing, and the passion that people develop for dancing over a period of time.

Dancing brings you tremendous joy, at the same time giving you many life prolongation benefits that enable you to live well into your old age in a healthy condition. It becomes a source of enjoyment, pleasure, exercise, fulfillment, mental growth, stimulation, social interaction and all-out fun that you can look forward to doing on a regular basis. When floating across the dance floor with a partner, you are connecting with another human being, in rhythm to the music, moving synchronously as if floating on air. So much for stress!

Dancing, as I will explain in the following chapters, is one of the best physical activities we can do to prolong our lives, prolong our enjoyment of life, and enhance our passion for living. *Dance to Live* is my gift to you. I hope you enjoy this book. Please pass it on to others so they may benefit from it and experience the wonderful feeling of dancing, too.

John P. Lenhart, M.D., D.C.
Saint Petersburg, Florida

Chapter 1

The Obvious:

Dance for Fun and Mood Elevation

Remember when you were a little kid. What did you do for fun? What gave you the feeling that you were really enjoying yourself? Was it running around with your friends, playing a game, being involved in an organized sport, or just hanging out with people having a good time?

If you go back and think about everything you did that was enjoyable, most of it involved doing something with somebody else, didn't it?

Generally, it's a lot more fun having fun *with* someone than by yourself—getting together with your best friend, or group of friends, and enjoying yourselves. Do you know what happens when you enjoy yourself?

Your endorphin levels rise.

Endorphins are those little hormones that make you feel good. They rise in your bloodstream when you're having a good time. They are little signals that you are feeling good.

I bet if you go back in your memory banks, you will remember the activity that you prepared for with great anticipation. You groomed yourself to look your absolute best in hopes of having that good time at a dance. A dance at a school, a church, a rec center, or at a friend's house—different venues called for different clothes sometimes—but these were the occasions when you looked forward to a good time. You smelled good and you looked great because you were going to try and impress the opposite sex.

You were on top of the world. That was your time to show off. It was an exciting moment. You were a little nervous, maybe, but you got over that as the music played and you got into the rhythm of the tune.

As the evening wore on, you became less and less inhibited and more prone to ask someone to dance; or if a girl, more willing to be available to be asked. It was an exciting moment in your life. The music, the activity, the social interaction made dressing up for the occasion worthwhile. You felt great.

Remember: That feeling of joy and excitement was brought on by Dance.

Dancing brings out the good in people. It makes them feel good and act good. It elevates their mood.

If you look good, you feel good about yourself. If you feel good about yourself, you act accordingly. Looking good, feeling good and acting accordingly translates to a great confidence level. And all of that can be achieved by dancing.

Dancing brings out the kid in you. It will allow you to be silly, act up, and do crazy things. You can become a ham. (There's a little bit of ham in all of us.) You can be creative. If you're really good, you can become the center of attention and everyone will watch you. And you'll feel good being looked at.

The music will allow you to express yourself, to move freely, to focus on the moods that the music is creating and let yourself go. Your mind will wander, the stress will disappear, and you will be totally engulfed in the rhythms of the music. You can express yourself any way you want in a safe environment and nobody is going to care because they are doing the same thing.

You can be fun loving and happy one moment, dancing to a fast song, and sexy the next, dancing to a slow song, enjoying the sensuality of the tune. And all this time you'll be touching someone.

Touch is therapeutic and dance is a safe environment in which to touch the opposite sex. It is a non-sexual, social process, in which people get to interact.

Isn't it wonderful to be able to go somewhere where everybody has the same purpose, which is to have fun and enjoy themselves. Dancing *is* fun. It is one of the best ways to enjoy yourself.

CHAPTER 2

The Importance of Physical Activity in Longevity

Now that you understand the reasons dance improves mood, discover something far more important and worth working on than just feeling good. Consider this:

PROBABLY THE MOST IMPORTANT SECRET OF **LONGEVITY** IS PHYSICAL ACTIVITY.

Physical activity, along with caloric restrictions, requires the greatest amount of self-control and self-discipline. Since I am a specialist in rehabilitation, this is a topic dear to my heart. I have produced twenty-eight specific rehabilitative exercise videos to restore joint mobility and strengthen surrounding muscles.

I also lecture to international physicians interested in alternative medicine in the anti-aging course at the American College for Advancement of Medicine. During my lecture, I ask everyone to stand and walk in place for the entire hour. I try to maintain a fairly steady pace and I count out the cadence for the doctors to walk in place. Periodically during my lecture, I look out to the audience to see how they are doing and urge them to keep up the pace.

There are many in the audience who are vigorous in their exercise efforts, some even jumping up and down from one leg to the other, raising their knees high to get the full benefit of the exercise. They continue that marathon effort throughout the entire hour.

However, after the initial fifteen minutes, and even more so after thirty minutes, a percentage of my audience stops exercising or greatly slows down. Mind you, these are physicians taking the course because they are interested in *anti-aging.*

How can doctors, proponents to be pioneers in alternative medicine and preventative medicine, be in such poor shape? Have they merely substituted vitamins for some drugs, or are they truly serious in making a change in themselves and their patients?

But you can't cheat nature. The rules of nature were laid down over millions of years.

You must be physically active to maintain joint function, muscle tone, mental acuity, hormonal function, and crucial metabolic pathways, including blood sugar transfer from our blood to our cells.

If you try to cheat nature, you cheat yourself.

If you remember nothing else, remember this:

Movement is life.

Every atom in the universe has movement. Even steel atoms have movement. Cells have movement. Nerve and muscle cells have movement. A brain wave pattern involves movements. Our thoughts involve movements, with transfer of chemical messages from one cell to another. The basic law of motion is universal.

Without movement, there is death.

And what is Dance except *Movement* with Music?

Right here I'd like to share with you some information and research that first appeared in my book, *7 SECRETS OF ANTI-AGING*. I feel these studies, which deal mainly with walking as a way of maintaining health and fostering anti-aging, apply also to the physical conditioning gained by dancing.

Babe Ruth, one of the greatest baseball players of the twentieth century, thought that life was like a bar of soap. You gradually wear it out until there is nothing left. In the era in which he lived, that made sense.

But, in the twenty-first century, it does not make sense because we know a lot more about human physiology. We know a lot more about nerve transmission and mental acuity. We know you can take a feeble, frail, nursing home patient in his nineties and within two months, rehabilitate his muscle strength and increase it by 174%. We know that. The baseball player didn't.

No matter how old you are, you can always improve your muscular performance significantly. Muscle cells *can* wear away like the Babe's bar of soap, but those same cells can be rebuilt, re-toned, re-strengthened. Your muscular strength and tone are directly related to your ability to be active when you are older.

Why did the eighty-eight-year-old ball player at the Kids 'n Kubs baseball field walk with a brisk pace, pick up a bat, and walk back to the dugout just like a forty year old?

Because he maintained his muscle tone and activity level. He was *continuously active* when he got older. In other words, he put in effort.

You have got to plan ahead. What you put in is exactly what you get out. There are no shortcuts. I know how hard it is to get out there and exercise three times a week; but I'll help you. At the end of this chapter, I'll give you the Lenhart Physical Activity Formula for Anti-Aging, derived after considerable research and analysis of hundreds of research articles, as well as personal experience through observation of patients and neighbors.

Sixty percent of the U.S. population is obese. Probably a greater percentage is inactive. Let's look at those statistics in economic terms. How many hundreds of billions of dollars have been made by the fast food industry to put on those wasted pounds? How many more billions were made by the biochemical industry to invent and process food so that it stays fresh forever, looks good, and tastes good? These chemists make a lot of money inventing chemicals to artificially fertilize the soil and kill all the pests in it, chemicals to grow food rapidly, and chemicals to preserve food and maintain its texture.

As a matter of fact, they are engineering pesticides to be built into the fertilizer so spraying of crops will not be necessary. Soon they will produce genetically altered beef and chicken with feed that produces huge quantities of hormones. The animals will grow faster and slaughterhouses will become more profitable.

Let's continue the economic aspect of your behavior further.

Due to your poor lifestyle habits, the medical industry will get larger and larger. Baby boomers grew up on fast food, additives, chemicals, comfortable couches, easy chairs, high-fat and high-sugar munchies. As they age, drug companies and hospitals will make lots of money because those Boomers will need continual medical care.

Drug companies will compete at breakneck speed to create new magic pills to fight these diseases we have because of our poor lifestyles. The government will be near bankruptcy because of the high costs of Medicare and Medicaid to supply all the services to those who didn't take care of their bodies and minds and didn't plan ahead.

If you don't use it, you lose it.

If you sit back, relax, and do not put any effort into a preventive anti-aging health care program, you will suffer the consequences in the later stages of life.

Increasing your physical activity is the absolute cheapest, most efficient, most effective way to increase your life substantially, and at the same time, decrease all the diseases that plague us substantially in our older age. Physical activity done on a consistent, regular basis is, just by itself, the best anti-aging treatment available even without adding all the other possibilities mentioned in this book. The more physically active you become the greater you increase your odds for a healthier, disease-free, mentally alert retirement.

Dancing should become one of your main physical activities because it is so much fun.

About twelve years ago, I moved into a neighborhood in which one neighbor was a very elderly gentleman; at least, he looked very elderly. He was seventy-three-years-old, frail, pale, and walked real slow. I saw him start to go on short walks up and down the block on a daily basis. Eventually he started bike riding and increased his distance progressively.

Over the years as I watched this gentleman, I saw this old, frail person turn into a vigorous, strong, youthful individual. By the time he was eighty-five, he was walking at about a 3.5 mph pace in the morning and evening. If you saw him from the rear, not knowing how old he was, you would swear that he walked and looked like a forty-year-old. His legs had good muscle tone. He had a spring to his walk. He walked deliberately with a cadence and arm swing that one sees in younger people.[1]

The persistent, continuous physical activity that he made himself do not only caused him to recover, but it also caused him to grow biologically younger. It increased his stamina and kept him from developing many age-related diseases.

One day I asked him what else he did to keep himself so young and fit and he said he lifted weights on a regular basis to keep up his muscle tone.

I have since observed other individuals following a similar protocol of continued physical activity who were able to stay young well into their eighties and nineties. The people who danced, seemed to enjoy life more.

Why is maintaining physical activity so important? It is important because it preserves and strengthens your muscles, joints, ligaments, tendons, and bones. At the same time, it conditions your cardiovascular system and increases waste elimination. By pumping your muscles, you are forcing excretion of waste products that have accumulated. Increased cardiovascular stress due to the exercise conditions and strengthens your heart.

You may now be asking, "What does exercise have to do with conditioning your bones?" To tell you the truth, most doctors don't know either.

Usually only physicians who have studied radiology realize there is direct correlation of both growth and strength, which is directly proportional to the stress placed on the bone.

What is one of the most common disabilities that occurs in older individuals? Fractures of the hip and other bones. When people age, they don't stress their bones enough to make them strong. Any type of small trauma can cause the bone to break. When the bones break, people become immobilized. Then begins a downward cycle.

Immobility leads to muscle wasting. Muscle wasting leads to incapacitation. Incapacitation leads to further degeneration, loss of the ability to perform activities of daily living, and eventually, death.

How many people have you known who broke bones at an elderly age, never recovered, and rapidly thereafter, ended up dying?

Did you know that one week of bed rest causes you to lose twenty percent of your muscle mass. Every subsequent week of bed rest causes you to lose another twenty percent of the residual muscle mass. It does not take a mental genius to figure out how weak you can become in a very short period of time by not moving or stressing your muscles.

If you don't believe me, look at the astronauts. What happens after they return from space missions? Do they have to be helped out of their space vehicles? We've seen it many times. They come out frail, weak, and unsteady on their feet. That's because they didn't have the opportunity to stress their bones and muscles adequately enough in space.

It all goes back to the same rule. If you don't use it, you lose it—rapidly.

Let's get back to the bed rest patients. How long do you think it would take for them to regain their muscle strength? If they lose twenty percent of their muscle mass with one week of bed rest, in order to regain that, it would take maximum contraction of the muscles on a daily basis for one week to regain only ten percent of the muscle mass they lost. Now, they have to do this for every muscle group that has been weakened. That's a heck of a lot of work to regain ten percent.

Think of it: You lose twenty percent of your muscle mass with one week of bed rest, but you can regain only ten percent of your muscle mass at maximum work of every muscle group. That doesn't seem fair does it, but that's the way biology works.

You must continue to use your muscles, ligaments, and tendons and put stress on your bones to maintain function and prevent disability.

In this chapter, I will get into some of the basic research data to back up some of my statements. If you look at the Kids 'n Kubs 1998 World Champion Baseball Team in St. Petersburg, whose members were all over eighty, you'll see that they maintained a joyful, physical-activity-filled retirement. They continuously moved their bodies, stressed their joints, ligaments, and tendons and constantly maintained muscle tone, which preserved the joints, bones, and overall health.

Going back to my rehabilitation literature, let's go over what happens to your body with inactivity. Let's see how many diseases you will recognize simply due to immobility. By explaining to you the body's responses to immobility, you will be able to determine the beneficial effect of physical activity almost immediately because the effects of immobility and inactivity are just about the same as the effects of aging.

Your central nervous system, which is the electrical system for your body, reacts to immobilization by decreasing your sensations. It decreases your ability to move. Your motions change, as well as your behavior, and you start to lose intellectual ability. In other words, you cannot think as clearly.

Your muscular system, which makes all your bones move and gives you propulsion, allows you to stand, breathe, sit, and walk, not only loses up to twenty percent of its initial strength during one week of bed rest, but with immobilization, the endurance decreases, the muscles atrophy, and you lose coordination.

What about your bones? I mentioned before that bones react to the stresses placed upon them. With immobilization, you get osteoporosis. You've heard of that. Osteoporosis is thinning of the bone, which leads to fractures, which leads to disability, which eventually leads to death.

You also get fibrosis. This means you get scar tissues forming at your joints causing them to eventually fuse so you cannot move. Well, that's a bummer. If you can't move, you're in a dying state because the reverse of dying is movement.

Then there's your cardiovascular system, your heart and circulation. With immobility, your heart rate is increased. Your blood pressure drops when you stand up or sit up, causing you to pass out. You also get blood clots. Blood clots lead to inability to breathe and suffocation, or, if they go to the brain, you have a stroke.

These things happen because you are not moving. You also get what is called a decreased cardiac reserve. The heart just cannot pump as well to get the blood to the vital organs and muscles.

What about your breathing? What happens to your breathing if you get immobilized? Well, you can't breathe as well. You cannot take in as much air because of what is known as a restrictive impairment. You're not getting as much oxygen because there is less oxygen going across your membranes and you need oxygen to live. One of the worse things that happens is you can't cough as much.

So, what's the big deal?

Well, just think about it. We have to cough to get junk out of our lungs. If we accidentally aspirate something or if we have a cold, or if we just have mucous building up in our lungs, we have to be able to cough to move it out. If you cannot cough, you'll get a major infection, and you die because the lungs fill up with fluid. That increased fluid is a great opportunity for bacteria to set in and give you pneumonia and fever, which can lead to death; or worse, a virus gets in there and you get viral pneumonia which we cannot treat with antibiotics. Unless you have great resistance, which you don't because you are immobilized and not moving, you will most likely die. All because of something that is preventable for the most part.

How about your digestive system? You lose your appetite and become constipated. What about your kidneys? You end up peeing more. You end up losing some of your sodium, which is very important for your body. You end up losing calcium. That explains why you become osteoporotic; calcium is taken out of your bone. You end up getting kidney stones, which are extremely painful.

What about your skin? The skin starts to atrophy. Atrophy is a wearing away or thinning of the skin and you end up getting bedsores. Bedsores lead to big ulcers, which lead to infections—it is a really messy situation.

What I have described to you is how the systems in the body break down *just by immobilization and inactivity.* If you look at older, frail, immobile individuals, you will see the same symptoms I described. It is a cascade of events. One thing leads to another, to another, until eventually the person dies.

Let me give you an example of the oldest man in Japan. He lived in Okinawa, an island noted for high nutrient foods, low calorie, restricted diets. He reached 112-years-old. He did agricultural work until he was eighty-five. That means he was doing hard, physical labor to keep his muscles and joints moving.

He remained active after he stopped doing farm work. He was a Type A personality, very active mentally and physically. His blood tests were normal. He was able to take care of himself completely until he was 108-years-old when something happened to him and he had to go to a hospital. Well, guess what happened?

Once he got to the hospital, he lost control of his life, his individuality and movements. What happens in a hospital? Immobilization. He deteriorated rapidly and in three years, went from normal to dementia.

This is a good example of what immobility does to you in a very rapid succession, especially if you are older.

What about immobility of the brain? The Use It or Lose It principle holds true in all the systems of our body. Your ability to think clearly and make decisions rapidly is based upon the number of connections you have in your brain called dendrites. Dendrites are like small branches in an oak tree that fan out and give the tree its shape. Those things talk to each other.

Let's assume you have a dense forest with a lot of these trees with the branches intermingling because they are so tightly packed. The more of these branches you have, the more they are going to intermingle.

Let's say you have a small monkey jumping from one branch to another, and a bigger monkey is chasing him. The more of these little branches intertwine between the trees, the faster he'll be able to run away and make a connection from one tree to the next and elude his predator and the faster will be his forward progress.

In other words, his forward progress will be unimpeded.

However, if the trees had few branches and they were further apart, this little monkey would have great difficulty jumping from one tree to the next because there would be fewer branches available for him to grab. His progress would be slowed and he will have a greater chance of being caught by the larger monkey and possibly eaten.

Your brain gets eaten if you don't have those dendrites.

There was a study done on rats placed into a playpen for an hour a day where the objects varied every day. They got to run around and constantly explore new environments. It was a very intellectually stimulating experience for the rats. Plus, a physically charged experience because they had to crawl up and down and around all these objects.

Another group of rats didn't get the exercise and were not put into this mentally challenging environment for an hour a day.

At the end of the experiment, the rats were sacrificed and their brains studied. Guess what they found?

The brains that were physically and mentally challenged had a large number of connectors (dendrites), like the sprouting branches of a tree, which are evident in very young people because they still have to learn a lot of new things. The rats not physically and mentally stimulated had considerably fewer connectors, fewer branches to make connections. That's similar to older people who are not mentally challenged.

You see, people used to think, just like the old bar of soap I mentioned before, that generally, your brain just wears out, deteriorates, and shrinks in size. If you take MRIs of people's brains, you will see atrophy in older individuals. There is a lot more fluid and a lot less gray matter, which is the stuff that does the thinking. However, it does not have to be that way.

There is a group of researchers studying nuns in Mankato, Minnesota. They live in a convent and routinely live past their nineties. These nuns were progressive educators, so they donated their brains to science after they died, a noble cause.

It was discovered that the college educated ones lived longer and because the religious order believed that an idle mind is the devil's playground, the nuns constantly did brain exercises—crossword puzzles, playing Jeopardy on television, constantly stimulating their minds to think. On autopsy, they found the nuns all had extensive brain dendrite formation at the time of death due to the intellectual stimulation. In other words, they were mentally young. The researchers noted that the ones who stayed mentally active did not suffer from dementia as much as those who didn't.

Newer research is also finding that people who have lost some of their intellectual capacity can regain it by constantly stimulating their brains. They can actually grow new dendrites, not just keep the ones they have, which is a very, very encouraging finding.

You can grow intellectually younger just by stressing your brain and making it work, constantly teaching it new things. It is the old Use It or Lose It philosophy.

The more I started thinking about this, the more I started thinking about my own life, how I am constantly changing and learning new things. There must be some kind of hidden signal telling me that it is time for me to become intellectually challenged again. Once I have learned one topic and used it for a while, I tend to move on to another field of medicine or business or computer science that stimulates my intellect. I also like working on several things at the same time with different intellectually stimulating capacities.

Every different thing you do stimulates a different part of your brain.

Going back to the Darwinian theory of evolution—Darwin was the guy who did all of his research in the Galapagos Islands off the coast of Ecuador where he discovered different birds developed in different ways and became highly specialized in food gathering and that is why they survived. He had a group of finches that were divergent; they could eat different types of seed and survive in different environments. Others could eat only one type of seed. If that plant became extinct, that species also became extinct.

Your brain works in the same way. It has to have a large variety of stimuli to keep it going and keep it growing. If you develop only one certain aspect of your brain, the other aspects tend to wither away because they're not being used and not being stimulated.

You become one-sided and, as your spouse may think, boring. I hate to say this, but people who only talk about one thing, know one thing, work at one thing are not as interesting as people who know a lot about a lot of different things and can hold a variety of conversations on an intellectual level. A quest for knowledge is one of the most enduring qualities a human can have. That is what differentiates him or her from other mammalian creatures, such as apes.

Let's summarize this subject by reminding you that the more connectors you have, the better is your ability to make connections. It holds true in the business world just as much as in your brain. The second part to this is that intellectual stimulation can cause dendrites to branch out, creating networks of new connections. Use It or Lose It.

Muscles. What do muscles do? It seems obvious. They hold up your skeleton, protect your organs, and provide movement to the bony part. They must be used constantly to maintain performance and keep you alive. If you don't believe me, look at people suffering from muscular dystrophy. You've seen the telethons on television about muscular dystrophy, but you probably never fully realized what that disease does. It slowly destroys your muscles until they wear out. When the muscles wear out, you can't even sit in a wheelchair. After awhile, you can't breathe, and you die. That is how important your muscles are. Your heart is a big muscle.

Bones. Bones provide a framework, something to attach things to, such as does your house foundation and outside walls. They provide structure. They hold things up. They are attachment points for muscles. They facilitate movements through joints. They allow the joints to move in and out or in circles or whatever different joints in your body do, or talk, as I'm doing right now dictating this book. However, in order for those bones to work properly and not break and fall apart, they need stress to maintain their mineral content and the honeycomb patterns inside the bones that give it strength.

Bones have a honeycomb structure inside them that is kind of a grid like, as used on the Eiffel Tower in Paris, a grid work of iron put together that reinforces one piece to the next and gives it strength. Bones do the same thing. If you don't stress these bones, if you don't move the bones and constantly use the bones, they lose that grid work.

When you lose some of that grid work, what happens to the structure? It weakens. Just think if you took half the supporting structures out of the Eiffel Tower and a big wind came along. Do you think the Tower would stay standing or do you think it would collapse? The same thing happens to your bones.

You have to use them. You have to stress them in order for them to keep on building new bone and creating new supporting structure, called the trabeculae.

Bone is constantly reinforcing itself by any stress put on it to make sure it is the strongest to bear that weight. So, fat people gradually get stronger bones because they have more weight to carry. However, there is a down side to it: The bone joints cannot bear the weight as easily so they wear out.

Bone joints are made of cartilage and cartilage does not rebuild itself as easily as bones do to accommodate the stress placed upon it. Large people develop bad knees and bad joints because too much stress is placed upon those joints. However, if these joints are used constantly and lubricated through motion, there is less chance of them wearing out and greater chance of new layers of cartilage forming over the joint. Dancing will lubricate those joints and help rebuild those cartilage layers.

There was a study done of a one-year walking program for women. What they found was that over that one year they had an increase of calcium in the top of the hip joint. However, there was no increase in calcium inside the wrist bones. Since women are prone to hip fractures, it showed that walking increased the strength of their hips. However, because the stress was only placed upon the hip joints and not the wrists joints. The extra bone deposits were placed where the stress was placed— in the hips.

So, what are the benefits of healthy bones, muscles, and ligaments?   You get movement without impediment or disease. You get movement without pain. Isn't that wonderful? You prevent bone damage. You prevent muscular or ligament destruction.   You gain power, speed, mobility, freedom, and a greater quality of life. You prevent debilitation and death. Use It or Lose It.

You may be saying, "That's fine, but I'm ninety. I didn't know about all your data. I didn't read this book till now."

I have good news for you.   A group of ninety-year-olds sitting around in a nursing home with nothing to do agreed to participate in a strengthening program. They did eight weeks of high intensity resistance training. The age group was eighty-seven to ninety-six.   They trained one muscle group, the quadriceps, which is in the front of your thigh.   In just eight weeks, they found increased strength of 174%. ONE HUNDRED AND SEVENTY-FOUR PERCENT IN JUST EIGHT WEEKS!

By strengthening that one muscle group, their walking speed increased by 48%. *These were eighty-*

seven to ninety-six year-olds! They were able to rebuild their muscle mass and regain strength by 174%. To me, that is remarkable. It tells me that Use It or Lose It' does not necessarily mean lose it forever. You can regain it.

Remember, movement is life. If you regain your muscle strength, you regain movement, you regain freedom, and you regain your quality of life.

Take a look at John Glenn, a retired astronaut. When he was seventy-seven years old, he returned to space. NASA scientists said he handled the rigors of space every bit as well as astronauts half his age. He suffered no more bone mass loss or muscle loss than the younger astronauts. His heart rate before, during, and after the flight was actually better than the average of twelve younger male astronauts. Isn't that amazing? The message is clear.

At seventy-seven you can do as well as a forty-year-old astronaut.

Glenn walked several miles a day, which I believe is the main reason he did so well. He also does some weight training and eats a balanced diet. Dr. David

Williams, director of NASA's Life Science Division and a former shuttle astronaut himself, stated that Glenn challenged the widespread notion that all seniors are frail individuals.

John Glenn did just as well as his younger counterparts. He spent four nights in a wired-up sleep suit. He provided seventeen blood samples and wore a small data recorder for twenty-four hours to monitor his heart rate. He also swallowed a capsule holding a radio transmitter and temperature sensor. How much more evidence do you need to see that at just about any age you can become young again through physical activity. Glenn conditioned himself to the status of a young person. If he lost any functions, he regained them.

An interesting finding was that like all other astronauts, Glenn experienced some balance problems once he returned to earth, but he recovered just as quickly as the other astronauts, which surprised the scientists. Many elderly people have difficulty with balance.

You are never too old to start. Exercise improves circulation and cardiovascular life. It also builds and remodels bone and builds new muscle.

There is a study that measured the effects of physical activity and calcium intake on the bone mass of healthy women of different ages. Guess what they found?

If they took calcium alone, it had no effect on their bone mineral density. However, the people who exercised had a five percent increase in the bone mineral density in the exercised bones. Remember, I mentioned that you have to put stress on the bone in order for it to grow. However, there was no increase in bone mineral density in the non-weight bearing bones—the bones that were not exercised.

The older you are, the more benefits your bones have from exercise. Exercise of weight bearing bones builds mineral content, size, and strength.

Another important component of physical activity is that exercise decreases diabetes and reduces the risk of non-insulin-dependent diabetes. There are a number of studies showing the benefits of exercise on reducing the risk of diabetes.

With diabetes you have a higher blood sugar level. Normally there is a decline in insulin sensitivity associated with aging, inactivity, and obesity. If you lose weight and increase your physical activity, you will increase your insulin sensitivity and decrease your risk of diabetes. Diabetes is a chronic condition that greatly accelerates aging and often leads to premature death.

There was a study done in Finland with 898 men. The men were subjected to moderately intense physical activity at high levels of cardio-respiratory fitness. It was found that after four years the more active individuals had a reduced risk of non-insulin-dependent diabetes mellitus of forty-four percent. That is very significant. That is reducing your chance of diabetes almost in half just by increasing your physical activity. If you lose weight, you do even better.

They also took the overweight, high blood pressure people in this group who had a positive family history of diabetes and who were engaged in moderate-to-intense physical activity at least forty minutes a week. They reduced their risk of non-insulin-dependent diabetes by fifty-four percent compared to men who did not participate in such activities. What this is telling you is that the fatter you are, the more out of shape you are, and the more risk you have, the greater you will benefit from exercise. It is never too late to start a physically active program.

Another interesting thing that happens when you are physically active is you increase your growth hormone level. There was another study that measured the hormone levels, as well as the mineral levels and cardiovascular levels of endurance-trained postmenopausal women and sedentary women.

The endurance-trained postmenopausal women (probably greater than forty-five to fifty) had lower body fat, lower weight, and higher aerobic capacity. When normalized for weight, the bone mineral density was higher in the spine. The interesting part is the growth hormone level was increased.

"Well, that's fine, but I've abused my body for all these years. This isn't going to do me any good." You are wrong!

The more you abused your body in the past, the greater your benefits. It has been proven over and over again in numerous studies that people in terrible shape can greatly benefit from physical activity. As a matter of fact, they have the most to gain because they are the closest to the grave.

Some of the major impact studies I consider important were done at Harvard University, Harvard Alumni Health Study, Cooper Clinic in Dallas, Texas, a very well known aerobic and cardiovascular clinic, The Honolulu Heart Program, and in Finland, where they studied twins.

In the Harvard study, they took 17,321 men and studied them for approximately twenty-five years. They concluded that the men who were vigorously active had about fifteen to twenty-five percent less chance of dying. Physical activity also decreased coronary artery disease, decreased high blood pressure, decreased non-insulin-dependent diabetes, decreased colon cancer, and increased life. One of the findings was that only vigorous activity had the remarkable difference in prolonging life. You had to expend about 1500 calories a week. Of the 17,321 men studied, there were 259 deaths of vigorously active individuals and 380 deaths from the non-vigorously active individuals. That's a big difference. There was a direct relationship between total physical activity and mortality. What does that mean?

That means, the more active they were to a certain limit, the less chance there was of them dying. One hundred twenty-one more people died who were less active. That is almost one-third more deaths just because they were not engaged in physical activity.

At the Cooper Clinic in Dallas, Texas, they wanted to know if people who were initially in very poor condition could benefit from physical activity. They studied 9,777 men, ages twenty-two to eighty, with a five-year follow-up. They found, as expected, people who were fit in the beginning and end had the lowest death rate. However, the people who were unfit and became fit during the five-year follow-up study had a forty-four percent reduction of the risk of death. This included all causes of death.

This should hit you between the eyes like a sledgehammer. If you can decrease your chance of dying by forty-four percent, which is almost half, for all causes of death, wouldn't you jump on it?

I would go out and buy a treadmill and start walking every day, or just get a good pair of sneakers and start walking in a safe neighborhood. Wouldn't dancing be much more fun than walking? How much more proof do you need to get off your butt and get going? Are you going to spend all your money when you get older on doctors, hospitals, and nursing homes? It is your choice.

Remember, exercise pumps out toxins.   It prolongs life, and walking or dancing prolong life.

Let's get into the walking aspect. There was a study done in Honolulu of retired men by the Honolulu Heart Program. They took 707 non-smoking retired men from ages sixty-one to eighty-one, and did a twelve-year follow-up. They recorded the distance these people walked. What they found is the more miles a person walked per day, the less was the chance of dying.

The men who walked less than one mile a day died two times faster than those that walked two miles a day. Their death rate was 40.5% versus 23.8% for the ones who walked two miles a day. What does that tell you?

Based upon this study and other studies I have reviewed and lectured on, the magic number is two miles a day or more. Guess what else they found?

The most common cause of death in the sixty-one to eighty-one year old age group was cancer. The death rate for the people who walked less than one mile a day of cancer alone was 13.4%. For those who walked more than two miles a day, the death rate from cancer was 5.3%. That means those who walked less than one mile a day had twice the chance of dying from cancer than those who walked two miles or more per day. What a difference just one mile makes. Isn't that amazing?

That extra mile must trigger very important protective mechanisms in the body that keep your chemistry at balance, keep your body from going haywire, pumping out the toxins, increasing your cardiovascular fitness, increasing the oxygenation and nutrition to your cells.

Whenever I have a chance to learn from my patients about aging and longevity, I jump at the chance. Recently, I had a hair stylist who came in as a patient. I found out that she worked as a hair stylist in several adult living facilities, which I thought was quite a niche market for a beautician. I asked her about her observations of her older clients, questions primarily about their health, alertness, and what type of clients they made.

One interesting observation she told me was that the hundred-year-olds she does hair for are more active, walk better, and have a much better attitude about life than the seventy-five- to eighty-year-olds. She also said their minds and memories are better.

Another thing that came out is that the hundred-year-olds were more resilient. They could overcome setbacks better and were much more pleasant to deal with than the sickly seventy-five- to eighty-year-olds.

She said that the younger ones who were sickly, less active, and not as alert mentally always worried about things. They talked about negative things all the time, worrying that they'd break their hip someday. Don't you know, they do break their hips. The ones who are sick always talk about being sick. The optimistic patients never seem to get as ill. The older patients seem to live for the moment. They enjoy life and they overcome obstacles through a positive mental attitude and an active lifestyle.

That is an interesting observation because it mirrors exactly what I have been finding in my research and my own observations. The more active you are, the less time you have to worry. The less you worry, the less chances you will have of developing a physical ailment that can greatly debilitate you and lead you to an earlier grave.

There is no reason to constantly worry about your physical state because you can do something about it.

There was another study done at the Cooper Clinic in Dallas, this one involving 25,000 men and 7,000 women. Researchers wanted to determine how people benefit from physical activity regardless of the shape they were in when they started. The study lasted nineteen years. Low, moderate, and high fitness levels were established for smokers, people with high cholesterol, high blood pressure, and other health conditions.

They found: one, That low fitness was an important precursor to mortality, meaning the less fit you were, the greater your chance of getting ill; and two, That the protective effect of fitness held for smokers as well as nonsmokers, those with and without elevated cholesterol, and unhealthy and healthy persons.

Everyone benefited from increased physical activity. People with low cardio-respiratory fitness benefited, as did moderate and high cardio-respiratory fitness, as determined by smokers and nonsmokers.

Every category improved with fitness. Those with normal blood pressure, moderately high blood pressure, and high blood pressure all systematically improved after an exercise program. The same thing was true for people who were generally ill all the time.

Remember my neighbor I mentioned at the beginning of this chapter, how I first met him when he was in his seventies? When I moved out of the neighborhood, he was well into his eighties and was in better shape than he'd been in his early seventies. The same observation I had on this one subject was observed at the Cooper Clinic with 32,000 subjects, which is the same observation my hair stylist patient noticed in her adult living facility centurions. Dance instructors notice a remarkable transformation in their elder students.

By the way, did you know exercise also decreases breast cancer by twenty to thirty-three percent? There are a couple of studies done about three years apart, one in

Norway and another in the United States, which came up with these conclusions. Wouldn't it be wonderful if you could decrease your breast cancer chances just by dancing?

No matter what you say, some people will also be skeptical. You know why—because they don't want to put in the effort. They think they are doomed. They think it is in their genes. They say, "Whatever happens, happens. I was destined to have cardiovascular disease...or cancer...or diabetes...." They just give up.

I knew there would be objections to my findings, so I dug deep in the literature and found a study done in Finland, which was titled, *Relationship of Leisure Time, Physical Activity, and Mortality the Finnish Twin Cohort Study*. They knew that physical activity and fitness were believed to reduce premature mortality. What they did not know was if genetic factors modified this effect. (The, 'It's in your genes' hypothesis.) They went on to study twins. Twins are pretty much the same. They have the same parents, the same environment, the same food. Identical twins have the exact same genes because they come from the same egg.

In this study done between 1977 and 1994, they took 7,925 healthy men and 7,977 healthy women from ages twenty-five to sixty-four. They classified them into conditioning exercisers and sedentary people. The conditioning exercisers walked vigorously for thirty minutes at least six times a month. The other group had no leisure physical activity. (I consider thirty minutes six times per month nothing.) However, they considered that conditioning. Even with that minimal amount of effort, about one-and-a-half days a week of walking thirty minutes, the results of the twins where one died during the studied period showed the odds ratio for death was sixty-six percent for occasional exercisers and forty-four percent for conditioning exercisers.

That means the people who walked vigorously at least thirty minutes at least six times a month had a twenty-one percent less chance of dying than the occasional exercisers; and, this was in twin pairs just walking thirty minutes six times a month.

When all the results from all the twins were compared, adjusted for age and sex, you had a seventy-one percent chance of dying as often as a sedentary exerciser if you were an occasional exerciser, and a fifty-seven percent chance of dying as often as a sedentary person if you were a conditioning exerciser. You had a twenty-nine percent less chance of dying if you exercised occasionally and forty-three percent less chance of dying if you exercised vigorously. To me, those are remarkable figures.

Based upon the twins studied, if you exercise vigorously only six times a month for thirty minutes by walking, you reduce your death rate by more than forty percent. The overall conclusion of this study was that familial factors did not explain the mortality differences by physical activity found in an individual-based analysis. Occasional and conditioning twin exercisers had reduced risk of death compared to sedentary twins.

I think you should re-read that last line several times until it sinks in. One interesting finding in this study when I reviewed the raw data was that women seemed to do better than the men. If you took the sedentary women and let's assume they had a 100% chance of dying at the end of the study, the conditioning women had a twenty-four percent chance of dying. That means they reduced their chance of death by seventy-six percent just by walking vigorously thirty or more minutes six times a month. It's amazing. Absolutely amazing.

So wake up. The only thing that is keeping you from increasing your life span is you.

There have been other studies done that measure the benefits of lifestyle activity where they measured how active you were during the day. As expected, people who were more physically active during the day did better in their blood pressure, as well as in their body fat. What they are trying to show you is that it is not always necessary to have a structured physical activity program to get beneficial results from physical activity. However, the people in that group alone who did have a structured program had greater improvement in the cardio-respiratory fitness than those who were just more physically active in the daytime. So, you will get more benefit out of a structured program that you do on a regular basis.

Movement is life.

If you don't move, you die.

It is as simple as that.

You get progressive decomposition if you don't move due to lack of muscle and joint stress, which eventually leads to rapid death.

These statements above are extremely important because they wrap up in a nutshell exactly what happens to you if you are not physically active. If you do not have good muscle strength and coordination, you will trip and fall more and will not recover as easily

If your bones are weak because they have not been stressed, you break them more often, which will lead to further disability, bed rest, which can lead to pneumonia and eventual death, or you will have a greater chance of developing colon cancer, heart disease, and as shown in the Honolulu study, a fifty percent greater chance of developing all cancer just by not being physically active.

"Okay, okay. I've had enough data. Now tell me what to do." Here it is.

These are your options. There are different types of exercise:

1) cardiovascular/aerobic exercise; 2) strength building or bulking exercise like weightlifting with free

weights or machines; 3) load-bearing, such as walking, biking, or running; 4) rowing, which combines a lot of different type of movements; 5) you can be engaged in sexercise. (Did you know there was a study that men who have more orgasms live longer? I'm not making this up; it was an actual study.) Another form of exercise I think is really good is tennis; 6) Golf-walking is a good form of exercise as long as you don't ride the cart. A golf swing, however, is not the best thing for your low back. 7) Skiing, such as cross-country and down hill is a good form of exercise. 8) Swimming has been a favorite exercise of mine for a number of reasons. It promotes range of motion throughout all your joints and it helps in resurfacing your joints as they become arthritic; 9) Dancing is one of my favorite exercises because it reduces stress and promotes joint movement. At the same time you are moving and having fun, you are building up new bone, strengthening your bones at the same time, reducing the risk of fractures as you will see in the following chapters. It can be a great social experience and you can do it well into your nineties. I saw an article recently about a ninety-eight-year-old woman in Naples, Fla., who still dances several times a week. She was in great shape physically and mentally enjoying life one day at a time.

You should move as much as you can and reduce the stress on your joints by weight maintenance. Caloric restriction is one of the better ways to do it. That alone will increase your life.

You should exercise your mind and body at the same time that you eat less. If you do that, you'll live longer and know that you are living. If you stress your body through exercise, give it proper nutrients, and reduce your caloric intake, you'll have a better balance in the body's chemical reactions. Your body and mind will give you much better service.

Remember the studies I quoted with the rats who were mentally stimulated and the nuns who were mentally stimulated well into their nineties and had brains of young people, and the ninety-year-olds who increased their muscle strength by 174%. All of this is possible. And don't forget our astronaut who performed as well as forty-year-olds after his space flight.

Everything is possible if you get moving. What did Jack LaLane, the old guru of exercise, say? When he wrote his book at the age of eighty-three, he said, "Old age is always twenty years away." He also stated, "There ain't no fountain of youth. What you put into your body is exactly what you get out of it." How true that is.

And it is true in everything. What you put into your life, you get out. How you make your bed is exactly how you will sleep on it. What you sow is exactly what you will reap.

Now for the Lenhart exercise program for longevity.

I came up with this formula after reviewing hundreds of articles on physical activity from the lectures I give to physicians who take the anti-aging seminars. If you follow these examples, you will greatly, greatly increase your chance of living longer and healthier, as well as knowing that you are living by staying mentally alert and continuously stay excited about life.

1. Pump iron for 15-minutes a day to discomfort. That means, lifting various types of weights to stress your muscles.

2. Change the muscle group each time you weight train. That means, change the muscles you are exercising. If you are doing certain upper body exercises one day, you do different upper body exercises the next day or lower body exercises. It is not that difficult with free weights to cover most of the muscle groups in the body.

3. Walk three miles in forty-five minutes or to a good sweat. Why is that important? You have to walk to a pace that actually stresses your body to a certain extent. You have to sweat a little but not a lot. Just so you are slightly clammy. Sweating helps release toxins through the pores in your skin. It also builds up your cardiovascular fitness by increasing your heart rate and increasing your oxygenation.

4. Use comfortable shock-absorbing walking shoes to reduce the ground reactive forces on your joints. One of the major problems people have with jogging or running is that they destroy their knees or ankles. I strongly recommend walking with cushioned shoes to

reduce joint stress that can eventually lead to osteoarthritis. I do not feel it is necessary to run to exhaustion and destroy your joints at the same time. All that is really necessary is to walk at a good pace to the point of sweating.

5. Smile and think happy thoughts while you are exercising. It is very important to have a good mental attitude and positive mindset most of the time, based upon my observations and the observations of others, and of the people who live to be very old. The ones who have the best mental attitude seem to do the best later in life.

6. Constantly stimulate your mind by learning new things and making your mind work. Your mental stimulation should also be varied, a diversity of interests and not limited to one thing. By dancing you get the benefit of walking as well as the mental stimulation of music and having to learn the dance steps.

7. Do the above exercise combinations at least three times per week.

Exercise is work, but the rewards are well worth it.

You will not only add years to your life, but you will add quality of life to your years.

As you can see from this chapter, movement is life. Without movement, you die. You can see from everything that I have written in this chapter, that it is extremely important for you to be physically active in order to live a healthy life.

One of the best ways to be physically active and greatly enjoy that activity is by dancing. Dancing will give you every one of the benefits I mention in this chapter. And on top of these physical benefits, you will have tremendous psychological benefits if you go out and dance. Believe me, I have seen it work for many, many people. Just go out and do it.

Note: This chapter was modified from my *7 SECRETS OF ANTI-AGING* book. I felt that it was important to present in this book, the research done on physical activity in my previous book.

As you will see in future chapters, dancing not only brings you the tremendous rewards mentioned in this chapter but it also gives you social and psychological rewards that far exceed the physical longevity benefits.

This original chapter can be read on my web site *www.antiagingrevolution.com.*

CHAPTER 3

Dancing for Joint Preservation

What are joints? Have you ever thought about that? We all seem to take them for granted, but they are essential in movement for our skeletal system. The only way a joint can move is if a muscle attached to either end of the joint, causing it either to bend, glide or rotate. Joints are areas where two bones come together and move in different directions. The direction of the movement of the bone is predetermined by the muscles attached to the bone.

If you look at your arm, you will see there are muscles above and below your elbow. In order for your arm to bend, the muscles above the elbow, such as the biceps femoris, have to pull up the bone below the elbow. It is not a very efficient system because if you were to design a machine that did the same thing, you would attach a muscle at the shoulder region and attach a muscle at the hand region, just tighten it up, and you would get a tremendous amount of power through your elbow joint. But that is not how the body is designed.

The muscles above the elbow attach just below the elbow, and they have to create a tremendous amount of force to get the elbow to bend. It is a very inefficient level system. As the elbow bends, it creates stress on the joint between the upper arm and the lower arm because the two bones are pushing against each other in order to stay in alignment.

In order to protect the bones, the joint, or union of two surfaces, is protected by a cartilaginous substance, which absorbs the forces of the two bones rubbing against each other. With excessive force or improper alignment, you can wear out those protective cartilaginous surfaces and end up with a situation where bone pushes against bone.

That situation is called <u>osteoarthritis</u>.

Osteoarthritis is generally known as a wear-and-tear condition, either due to overuse or improper use of a joint surface. The natural reaction of a body in osteoarthritis is to form excess bone around the joint. In X-rays, that excess bone looks like little spurs around the joint surface. It is these little spurs that cause pain.

The pain you get from those little spurs causes you to become immobilized trying to protect the joint, which in effect causes you more harm.

The immobility of a joint leads to fibrosis and ankylosis of a joint. What do those two terms mean?

Fibrosis means fibers develop around the joint, preventing it from moving very much. *Ankylosis* means the joint fuses. And what good is a joint if it is fused? You can't move it. So you lose range of motion of that joint, becoming further immobilized.

A joint becomes fibrosed or ankylosed to varying degrees if it is not subjected to active or passive motion. That means that joints have to be moved in order to keep them from being fused. When that happens, the muscles around the joint are gradually replaced by connective tissue.

This connective tissue makes the joint very stiff and unable to move. Because of this excessive buildup of connective tissue, the joint may become deformed, which in turn makes it much more difficult to move. The deformed joint with excessive amount of fibrotic tissue around it, eventually becomes calcified. This calcification is called ectopic calcification of the soft tissues surrounding the joint. This calcification, calcium buildup around the joints, may cause permanent fusion, also known as ankylosis of that joint.

There are many types of joints in the body. The example I gave was an elbow—a hinge joint. There are also joints that rotate, such as your shoulder joint, or ball and socket joints, such as your hip.

Did you know, that in your spine you have 24 bones above your pelvis? Each one of those spinal bones has six joints to it, which cause each segment of the spine to move. These joints primarily have a gliding motion, or do rotation.

Nevertheless, there are six joints to every one of your spinal bones. If you add that up, that is a total of 144 joints just in your spine, between your neck and your pelvis. Add to that the 12 ribs which also attach to your spine and form joints with your spine, you have a total of 156 joints surrounding your spine above the pelvis. That's a lot of joints where things can go wrong.

If you look at your wrist, there are eight individual bones inside it that form joints, which allow your wrist to bend, go backwards, go sideways, or rotate. I think you get the point. The body has many joints and every one of those joints has to be moved.

If they aren't, they eventually rust in place and you will not be able to use them. Take for example, hinges. If a hinge to a door or a gate is left unused, eventually rust will develop and the rust will lock the hinge shut. Think of the joints of your body as hinges. Those hinges need to be constantly moved. In a door hinge, you can always squirt some oil on it, move it a little bit and get it going. But in a human body joint, there is no way you can squirt oil in it to get it going.

The only way a joint is lubricated is by usage.

There is a fluid inside the joint called *synovial* fluid. This fluid bathes the joint and keeps it lubricated. The only way to replenish that fluid is by constant movement.

It is much easier to keep a joint moving than to repair it later on when it is all calcified.

Dancing is a great exercise to preserve your joints because it is low impact. Aerobic exercise or running will cause jarring motions on your joints. These jarring motions can lead to arthritis. Walking and dancing, however, create gliding motions, and gliding motions are joint enhancing because they stimulate the pumping of the synovial fluid for lubrication and they also stimulate joint cartilage growth and repair. Gliding, low impact joint motion, is the best motion you can possibly do to rehabilitate your joints and preserve them.

After knee surgery, many orthopaedic surgeons put their patients on active/passive motion machines. Those machines do continuous motion of the joint in order to stimulate healing and joint preservation—the same thing you do when you dance. I have seen many people, well into their late 80's and 90's, who have excellent joint health because they dance on a regular basis.

CHAPTER 4

Dancing for Bone Strengthening

Did you know that bone is a living organism that constantly changes its makeup? Bones react to the stresses placed upon them. If you don't put any stresses on your bones, they will become frail and brittle, and they will break very easily.

As a specialist in orthopaedic medicine, I can tell you the patients who put stress on their bones by either walking on a regular basis or dancing, have much stronger bones than the patients who spend all of their time in sedentary activities, such as watching television. You can see this difference by looking at X-rays. The X-rays of patients who exercise on a regular basis have a much healthier appearance.

On a recent study funded by NASA to test how long periods of immobilization affected bone, they found that non weight bearing conditions acted to impair cortical bone fracture healing by having less functional bone progenitor cells at the repair site. These progenitor cells are required to heal bone fractures. When you break a bone, there is a callus that forms around the fracture site that surrounds the fracture and brings in new bone cells. This callus becomes very hard and strengthens the bone as it heals. What they found in non-weight bearing conditions was that the callus around the fracture site was very poor in its quality. It had a decreased size and was more brittle. When they examined this callus, or this bony deposit around the fracture site, they found that there was inadequate mineralization of the extracellular matrix, which is the bone composition itself around the fracture site. This decreased mineralization causes the bone to be very frail and have a tendency to break again. When the number of cells, called, connective tissue progenitor cells, were counted around the fracture site, they found there were only 24% as many cells in a non weight bearing bone in contrast to a weight bearing bone.

Therefore, extended immobilization leads to failure to heal long bone fractures.

The failure to heal occurs because there are fewer cells present. Fewer cells making bone means weaker bone. This study greatly backs up the premise of "use it or lose it."

This premise exists in every aspect of our body from our brain to our joints to our bones. If you sit around and are immobile, there is absolutely no reason for your bone cells to work hard and do their job, which is to make strong bones. The older you are, the more important it is for you to have strong bones, because it is a lot easier to break a bone at an older age than at a young age.

Let me tell you a little story about a friend of mine who is 89, whom I have known socially through dancing.

This lady had continuously danced most of her life, and had outlived her husband and a subsequent boyfriend. Three months ago I heard that she had broken her hip after taking a terrible fall off a sidewalk. I felt sorry for her because I knew she loved to dance so much, and having a broken hip would keep her from dancing.

Last week, at a local club, I was surprised to see her at an adjacent table setting, and when she got up to go on the dance floor, I was even more surprised. After all, her hip fracture and hip replacement were only two months ago. When she finished dancing, she came to my table and started talking, and told me about how she fell and broke her hip and so on, and how dancing has enabled her to heal much more rapidly, and become active again.

I asked her to dance, and to my surprise, this lady could keep a perfect swing tune rhythm. She could also do a turn, at 89 with an artificial hip that was just replaced three months prior to this dance! It was amazing, simply amazing, how strong this woman's bones had become, simply by dancing.

There is a law in radiology and bone growth called the Wolff's Law, stating that the bone will directly remodel itself based upon the force applied to it. In other words, putting it in laymen's terminology, *the bone gets stronger only if it is stressed.* If you do not put stress on the bone, it becomes soft, weak, brittle, and subject to breaks.

The inside of a bone is a matrix, a criss-crossing matrix of cells. This matrix changes its position based upon the stress angles that are placed upon the bone. It always wants to buttress itself and strengthen itself according to the load placed on it. If you continuously place a load on the bone, the bone is going to become stronger and stronger. Strong bones have less tendency to break. Weak bones snap very easily.

If you put no stress on a bone, the bone will get weaker and weaker and weaker and the slightest amount of trauma will cause the bone to break.

One of the last things you want to break is a hip. A hip fracture takes you out of commission. It softens and weakens your bones because you are laid up for long periods of time. At the same time, it weakens your cardiovascular system and your muscular system and you become weak all over.

What's the solution to bone strengthening?
Dancing, of course.

Dancing is one of the best activities you can be engaged in for bone strengthening and bone preservation. It is a low impact activity that stresses your bones, making them stronger. The bones that become stronger are basically the leg bones and the hipbones as well as your spine, because that is where all the load bearing occurs.

Just the fact that you can strengthen your bones and help prevent them from breaking will greatly enhance your chances of living longer.

CHAPTER 5

Dancing for Cardiovascular Health

Your cardiovascular system refers basically to your heart, which in effect is a pump, and the miles and miles of blood vessels that this pump supplies. In order for this pump to work properly, it needs good nutrition and clean pipes through which it pumps the blood. The pipes, also known as blood vessels, either arteries or veins, feed oxygen and nutrients to every single cell in your body. The arteries are under a higher pressure because that is the blood that is coming directly from your heart to either your brain or to your arms, your gut and your legs. The veins are under less pressure, and they supply the blood that is returning to the heart after it has given up all its oxygen and nutrients to feed your cells.

It's a closed loop. The blood goes from your heart, through the arteries, to your muscles, bones, gut, and brain; it returns from your muscles, bones, gut and brain, to your heart to be pumped again into the lungs where the blood is oxygenated with rich oxygen that you breathe in, and returned back to the heart so that it can be pumped out again through your arteries to the rest of your body. This process gets repeated over and over and over again. The blood going to your gut, which is your intestinal system, comprising the small and large intestine, takes the nutrients that you absorb from your food and circulates those nutrients to the cells in the body. The cells use the nutrients for energy so they can do their job. If the cardiovascular system, your circulation, is clean, your heart doesn't have to work as hard. However, if your arteries are dirty and clogged, the heart has to work much harder to get those nutrients to your cells. If your arteries are clogged, they create more resistance in your blood vessels, and therefore your heart has to pump much harder to get the nutrition to your cells as well as the oxygen.

With immobility, you get increased heart rate. Your blood pressure drops when you stand or sit up, causing you to pass out. Blood clots are also a possibility. And blood clots lead to an inability to breathe and eventual suffocation, or, if the clots go to the brain, you have a stroke.

In addition, you develop what is called a *decreased cardiac reserve.* The heart just cannot pump as well to get the blood to the vital organs and muscles.

All that is a result *because you are not moving.*

As I said earlier, movement is life. Without movement, you die. As Einstein once said, *nothing happens until something moves.* Movement is life.

Your heart is constantly moving—beating, beating, beating—pumping that blood throughout your body, giving it nutrients that feed your cells and allow you to live.

You've seen people with purplish legs and feet and arms and fingers? These people have poor circulation. You see people all the time becoming short of breath when they climb one flight of stairs. You try to go for a walk with them and they can barely keep up with you. These people are deconditioned.

Maybe you are one of them.

You need to pump that blood to every little cell in your body. You need to give all those cells nutrients. You need to get oxygen. By increasing your cardiovascular efficiency, you will be able to keep yourself in good health.

Dancing is one of the best aerobic activities you can do to condition your cardiovascular system. You are exercising without knowing it. You are pumping the blood to every cell in your body. You are strengthening your heart muscle. You are allowing the smallest cells in your body to be fed with life giving oxygen and the nutrients they need. You are allowing your brain to have adequate oxygen, as well as the needed nutrients for it to function properly.

Dancing will condition your cardiovascular system without seeming that you are working. You could walk a treadmill every day or go and workout in the gym, but it is a lot more fun to go out there and dance several times a week and get the same thing accomplished without the drudgery of working out on some machine in the gym. You're having fun, you're listening to music, you're touching other people. Your endorphin level rises, and at the same time, your circulation improves and your heart rate improves and your heart efficiency improves.

And remember this: the faster the rhythm, the faster your feet will move, then the faster your heart will pump, and the more benefit your circulatory system will have.

Just by dancing—doing something enjoyable—your heart becomes much more efficient at pumping blood throughout your entire body. You slowly will condition yourself to greater and greater endurance. Before you know it, you will be able to walk further, you will be able to climb those stairs, and you are going to feel great.

I found that by dancing on a regular basis, I could spend less time working out. I felt better and my mind was clearer because of the fun I had dancing. And I could dance two to three hours without even feeling that I had exercised.

CHAPTER 6

Dancing and Weight Loss

Is there anything you hear more about today than the obesity epidemic in America? I don't think so. Fatness has pervaded society. There are many root causes for this, the most common one, inactivity. Past generations moved more. Physical labor, including such simple tasks as washing laundry, hanging it out to dry and then ironing it, have gone by the wayside for most Americans. Past generations walked more. They played more. And they ate better.

Can you imagine your grandparents going from house to car to office or store, reversing the procedure coming home, picking up fast food on the way, and then settling down on the couch for an evening of television? We've become a sedentary society at the same time we've become used to processed food rife with additives. It's no wonder fatness has become the norm.

And when we are overweight, *we don't like to move!*

Yet, once again I repeat: movement is life.

It is obvious in this chapter how dancing is beneficial.

Although there are overweight people who are good dancers, the stress put on the overweight person's heart and joints is not advantageous and in the long run can cause problems. If they are good dancers when hefty, think of their talents on the dance floor if they weren't carrying around all those pounds.

The calories burned during dancing are quite significant. For example, if you weighed 150 pounds, in a slow dance, such as a waltz or a fox trot, you would be burning approximately 220 calories an hour. Dancing disco or Latin or ballroom dances, you'd burn approximately 400 calories an hour. If you fast-danced, that number would go up to 430 calories per hour! If you weighed 175 pounds, in a slow dance you'd be burning 250 calories an hour and in a fast dance, you'd burning as much as 500 calories an hour. Not bad at all considering you've having fun.

The sustained movement of dance is an excellent low impact aerobic activity for weight loss. Dancing on a regular, consistent basis will shed those pounds regularly and consistently.

You will develop self-confidence and pride in yourself for what you have achieved. You'll feel good about yourself because you'll look better, and feel healthier because you'll be stronger and more agile than before.

CHAPTER 7

Dancing for Coordination Enhancement

Coordination and balance are so important as you get older, because they prevent you from having accidents. It is important to maintain your coordination and your responsiveness to things around you. Just think about it: you are driving your car and someone dashes in front of you. You need to be able to respond immediately and put on the brakes or swerve to the side to avoid an accident. You can't do that unless you have good coordination. You need to be able to recover from stumbles and slips and missteps without sustaining major damage to your body, such as broken bones and blood vessels.

All of these things depend upon your coordination.

Coordination may be defined as the ability to regulate multiple muscles simultaneously, or in sequence to perform apparently simple or complex activities. According to rehabilitation literature, you have to be able to combine various activities of a number of muscles into a smooth, coordinated pattern, so the contractions are in harmony with each other in order for you to perform a specific task. This coordination of muscle activity is the result of patterns that you have learned to perform a specific task. These patterns are learned early in your development, when you are learning to crawl, later on when you are learning to walk, and maintain your balance. What you are doing, in effect, is developing *engrams,* which are organized, preprogrammed patterns of muscular activity. You are stimulating certain muscles and inhibiting other muscles from contracting, resulting in a smooth action which looks flawless.

The development of coordination is totally dependent on repetition, just like learning is dependent on repetition. At first the movement is very simple, at a slow pace. Later on, the movements become more complex and the pace increases, just like in dancing.

When you repeat a particular activity over and over, an engram is formed, and you develop muscle memory, and the speed of that activity increases. With practice, you can perform that activity with little to no conscious effort, and it becomes automatic, or programmed.

To give you a very simple example, let's consider writing.

You have to learn how to make each letter, one at a time. It is a very arduous task. Once the engram is developed, you are able to write flawlessly and automatically. Because coordination is produced by repetition, it is lost through *lack* of repetition, or inactivity. It becomes necessary to re-teach coordination to muscles that have become inactive.

Only through specific training and repetition of a coordinated movement, do muscles again become normal in their activity. The more inactive someone is, the more uncoordinated they become. If you are sedentary, you gradually lose your coordinative abilities to respond to situations. You will more easily trip, be slower in responding to situations, and have a greater propensity to hurt yourself and become totally incapacitated.

When you learn to dance, you learn specific dance foot patterns and arm movement patterns. These patterns have to match the rhythm of the music which you are listening to. By combining the foot patterns that you have learned with the music that you hear, you automatically become more coordinated. These coordination skills you can take with you to all aspects of your life, be it sports, bicycling riding, or accident prevention. By improving your coordination, you are, in fact, tuning your nervous system to be more sensitive to specific movements. If you have trained your feet to be coordinated and your arms to act accordingly, you should be able to respond to other drivers much quicker and prevent accidents. Dancing may allow you to drive a car much longer in your life because you are more coordinated and you can respond quicker to adverse situations. Dancing is an excellent way to improve your response rate and enhance your coordination. By increasing your ability to respond to situations through improved coordination, you are reducing your chances of major injuries. If you can respond better to situations that can injure you, you will be able to live a healthier, safer life.

CHAPTER 8

Dancing For Muscle Growth and Toning

Muscles move bones. Muscles move blood through your circulatory system, and muscles give you mobility and the freedom to go from one place to another at will. Muscles are important in every aspect in the activities of daily living. You need muscles to breathe, you need muscles to propel the food through your digestive system, you need muscles for balance, and you need good muscles to be able to do things with your arms and walk. Good muscle tone is needed for simple things such as being able to stand up straight without falling over. When muscles start deteriorating because of lack of use, your whole body starts deteriorating to the point where it cannot function.

Muscles have to be used. They constantly have to be pumped in order to strengthen themselves and maintain their tone, as well as to grow. Look at weight lifters. The only way that they can grow their muscles and bulk up is by constantly pumping iron. They are using their muscles. They are forcing them to work hard. By doing that, the muscles grow.

Lack of use causes many things to break down. This is especially true of muscles. In *7 SECRETS OF ANTI-AGING,* I talk about an experiment done on 90-year olds in Hawaii, where sedentary retirees were put into an exercise regimen of several times a week, and within two months their muscle strength increased 175%.

You can increase your strength at any age. You can increase your coordination at any age, and you can increase your tone at any age. That's the beauty of using your muscles. If you use them, they will respond accordingly, and they will get stronger. Your balance will improve, your tone will improve, your stride will improve, and you will start acting younger than your age. If you are 30 years old, you will be acting like a 20-year-old; if you are 50 years old, you will be acting like a 30-

year-old; and, if you are 75 years old, you will be acting like you're 50. By increasing your muscle tone and strengthening your muscles by dancing, you will develop a faster stride in your walk and greater agility.

Let's go through the mechanics of dancing and how these mechanics increase your muscle tone and growth and help strengthen your muscles.

Dancing involves a rhythmic walking and sometimes, almost running. You are constantly going up and down on your toes and moving your upper body. You have to maintain a frame, which is a certain posture that has to be kept in a specific position as you go through your routines.

The act of maintaining a frame increases your muscle tone in the upper body, which includes your shoulders, arms and upper torso. Maintaining a frame also improves your posture. Often times, when you dance, your upper body frame remains at a fixed position while your lower body, your pelvis and your legs, are doing something totally different. You have to coordinate your upper body with your lower body whenever you go through a dance routine, in order for it to look good. This coordination of upper and lower body takes considerable amount of training in order to be executed properly. Just like an athlete, you are training your body to act according to the dance style that is being played, whether break dancing, free style rock and roll, a samba, a waltz, a cha-cha, a bolero, or a fox trot.

Each one of those dances requires a different rhythm and different coordination ability of your muscles. By doing a variety of dances, you are training your muscles and at the same time causing them to grow and become stronger.

Dancers have excellent muscle tone in their legs as well as in their pelvic and hip regions. If you watch Latin style dancers, you will notice that they have excellent coordination throughout their entire bodies, because all of their muscles have to act in synchrony to the rhythm that is being played.

The other day I went to the gym and started lifting weights and going through the machines and going on the rowing machine as well as the treadmill, and if I didn't have a partner to talk to, I would have been extremely bored doing that routine. On the other hand, if I go to a dance studio by myself, and interact with the other dancers, listening to the music and becoming engrossed in the rhythms of the music while I am dancing, I am receiving the same benefits of exercise that I get in the gym going through the stations.

I am preserving my joints, I am strengthening my bones, my cardiovascular system improves, I am able to lose weight, increase my coordination and strengthen my muscles at the same time. Best of all I am having fun while exercising. The music I am listening to while dancing is psychologically therapeutic and interacting with my dance partner through dance movement is socially and physically rewarding.

CHAPTER 9

Brain Growth and Memory Improvement

Prevention of Mental Deterioration

Dementia takes a long time to develop and is generally quite advanced when it is diagnosed. The protein amyloid clogs up nerve cells so that they cannot function properly. This clogging up of the brain with amyloid deposits leads to memory loss and dementia.

Lancet, a British medical journal, reported a study that occurred over twenty years and involved 1,500 men and women, 200 of whom developed dementia or Alzheimer's disease between the ages of 65 and 79. Those who developed Alzheimer's disease or dementia were far less physically active than those people who did not develop it.

The study found that you needed to be involved in physical activity to the point where you were breathless and sweating for 20 to 30 minutes, twice a week.

For healthy hearts and lungs, the recommendation was 30 minutes, three to five times per week.

Regular exercise will help keep the small blood vessels in your brain healthy and oxygenate your entire brain, in effect, preserving your memory. Exercise also reduces the protein amyloid, which clogs nerve cells as mentioned above.

Think of the ramifications of this most exciting study and the health benefits of dancing: If you exercise for at least half an hour twice a week during your midlife, such as in your 40's and 50's, you could significantly reduce the risk of dementia by as much as 50%. Those people prone to Alzheimer's disease could reduce Alzheimer's disease by as much as 60%. This is one of the first studies that show the effect of physical activity over a prolonged period of time.

In a recent study of nearly 500 people at the Albert Einstein Center in Bronx, New York, the researchers found that *dancing was the only regular physical activity that significantly decreased the dementia level in the subjects.*

It makes sense. In order to dance well, you have to concentrate on your steps and you have to remember your steps. You are exercising your brain at the same time that you are exercising your muscles. Studies on animals show that the connections between brain cells in rats and mice grew stronger and the neuron survival rate increased by increased physical activity.

And dancing is better for memory enhancement than other forms of exercise because of the social interactive factor.

The social interaction is an emotional support system that enhances brain development. Many years ago, studies done in psychology showed that apes that were constantly interacting as they were growing, thrived and developed rapidly, while apes that were not socially interactive, did not have touch and were isolated, even though they were given proper nutrition and physical activity, showed severe reduction in their development.

A study done at Rush Presbyterian St. Luke's Medical Center in Chicago, which was published in the *Journal of the American Medical Association* in 2002, compared a number of brain stimulating activities to see which had the most beneficial effect on vascular dementia, which is the most common form of dementia. The activities included reading, writing, board games, cards, discussion groups, music, puzzles, bicycling, swimming, dancing, and team sports.

The study concluded that dancing was the best activity to benefit the brain. This was because dancing involved social interaction as well as physical activity.

Researchers also found that frequency was important, and the more often you danced, the greater was the benefit for brain enhancement.

The process of having to memorize various dance steps and coordinate them to the music produces a continuous stimulation stream to the brain. The challenge of the brain in itself, along with the social interactive factor, causes the brain to grow more and become more active.

The brain is like a big muscle, the more you use it, the stronger it becomes. As we get older, we gradually lose the ability to remember recent events. They used to say, "You can't teach an old dog new tricks." That's because old dogs just laid around in the corner and did nothing. If these old dogs were made to run around and exercise every day, they certainly could learn new tricks.

By stimulating your brain, your memory retention of new events improves significantly. Dancing is a great mental challenge, which stimulates your brain to grow and greatly increases your chances to remember things. We remember things that happened many years ago, but the challenge is to remember things that happened recently. Dancing does a great job in improving that ability.

Whenever you are learning something and having fun at the same time, you will retain it much better than just having to do it for rote memory alone. Your brain gets a little bounce to it, when it learns something and has fun at the same time.

If you look at people walking down the street, some just kind of shuffle along while others have a cadence, where they sort of hop along and have a spirited walk to them. That is what happens to your brain. It gets a spirited jolt of stimulation that causes you to remember things better and causes your brain cells to stay active and grow.

Dancing is fun, challenging and socially interactive. It causes you to move to a certain rhythm, and stimulates the "feel good" centers in your brain, causing your brain cells to expand. And that makes you smarter.

CHAPTER 10

Dancing for Balance Improvement

Want to test your balance? Close your eyes and stand on one leg (you can extend your arms to your sides to keep from falling). How long can you stand without having to put the other leg down? Just for the heck of it, write down the date you first try this.

Generally, younger people can do it much longer than older people because our balance decreases as we get older.

Without balance we fall. When we fall, we can do a lot of damage to our body. It is really sad to see the number of people who fall in their shower, in their home, or just trip on the sidewalk and end up with a broken hip, in the hospital, and eventually dead.

Prolonged bed rest alone can kill you, because you lose so much muscle mass in the process. Your bones become demineralized and you develop osteopenia and osteoporosis. Your ligaments get weak and your overall strength decreases. You see why balance is so important?

You have to maintain your balance in order not to fall. You may want to take that balance test periodically once you get into your dance routine, just to see how much better you get. The better your balance, the less are your chances of injuring yourself from a simple stumble. You will be able to recover quicker if you do happen to stumble, and you will have fewer falling episodes, which can be devastating.

Now, why does dancing improve balance much more than any other type of physical activity, such as walking, running, bicycle riding or swimming?

Because dancing involves movement that is timed to rhythm.

The rhythm constantly changes, so your movement has to constantly change to keep pace with the rhythm. Sometimes you have to go fast, and sometimes you have to go slow, and sometimes you just have to stand in one position on your toes until the music changes so you can go fast again. These variations of balance, going up and down on your toes, stretching certain muscles to one direction and then to another direction and holding them in that position, causes you to train your muscles, your tendons, your ligaments, your bones, and your brain, not to fall. It tunes your whole body to be in balance.

Just the graceful floating motion of a waltz, with the up and down movements and the changes in direction improves your balance. Certain dances require rapid foot movements; other dances require torso movements, as you are gyrating your hips back and forth, trying to make it look good. Other dances require upper body movements, where you are moving your head in one direction and your shoulders and arms in another. All these are balancing movements that have to be counteracted by your lower body so that everything stays in alignment so that you don't fall. This training is phenomenal because it stimulates the balance centers in your brain. Constant stimulation of those centers causes them to get better and better and better, and what happens? You don't fall. *Not falling* is a good thing.

Recently I went to an 18-piece big band dance at a local club, and a friend of mine said, "There is So and So; she's a former associate of Arthur Murray."

This lady must have been 80-some years old and she was thin, walked upright and erect, and had phenomenal posture. Her shoulders were back, and she had a great presence to her. She owned a dance studio and was associated with this famous dance instructor—I've got to dance with this lady, I thought to myself.

So I went up asked her to dance. She stood up right away and was happy to dance with me. She perked up when she started to dance, as if a new person was born that came out of her and the enthusiasm was there. You could just see it in her facial expression and her body movement.

But you know what surprised me? *She had perfect balance.* She didn't sway, she didn't hang on to me. She maintained her posture, her stance, and the rhythm as she balanced herself through the various movements I put her through.

Dancing the rumba, she not only went through the rumba steps, she also put hip motions and gyrations into the dance itself. Now those are hard moves to do and still make them look good. Yet here was a woman well into her 80's, who *still* had great rhythm and phenomenal balance.

Dancing is self-preservation, which is fun. How many things do we do in life that have phenomenal health benefits and at the same time we have a great time doing them?

Yes, my friend, we can dance to live. And, after a while you will live to dance, because you will have so much fun doing it. Someday you'll wonder how you lived without it.

CHAPTER 11

Dancing For Stress Reduction

Where does stress come from? Worry. And who doesn't worry? After all, there are often times when things seem out of our control (and sometimes they really are), so who wouldn't worry? Problem is, worry is the oxymoronic *impotent energy*. It takes energy to worry but the energy expended doesn't solve anything, so we become tired and stressed.

Stress causes cortisol levels in our blood to rise and high levels of cortisol are destructive to our bodies.

The hormone cortisol is important to your body because it is released when we are in an excited state, such as when we are about to flee from a predator or a dangerous situation, and we need a quick burst of energy to run very fast. At that time our sensitivity to pain is decreased because all we are worried about is our survival. We can develop almost superhuman strength and be able to flee from fearful situations. Cortisol generally occurs in short bursts in our body, and helps us to avoid dangerous situations and heightens our senses, and gives us that extra burst of energy we need to avoid predators. Cortisol is often very high in people involved in battle. It creates a hyper-excited state.

What do you think happens if you chronically increase the cortisol level because of chronic stress? Well, you can develop all kinds of conditions, such as elevated blood sugar, decrease in your muscle strength, high blood pressure, lowered immunity, increased fat in your belly. You can even have weaker bones. Your thyroid may not function as well, and you may have the inability to think clearly. When you are chronically stressed out, you set off a series of events in your body that gradually and slowly destroy you.

Recently cortisol has been associated with the obesity epidemic we have in our country, because our society seems to be chronically under stress. People are always worrying about something, or having to run from one place to another just to stay even, and not drown under a mountain of debt and the increased amount of pressure that is put upon us just to live in today's modern society.

In a recent article which studied bed rest and cortisol induced stress, there was a three-fold greater loss of lean body mass and a 50% greater loss of muscle strength after 28 days of bedrest. We know that inactivity, or bed rest alone, can destroy muscle mass, but if you add stress on top of that, you have a much greater destructive effect on your body than just bed rest alone.

Memory can be significantly reduced by elevated levels of cortisol. Cortisol is increased in your system with physical stress as well as psychological stress. The problem occurs when the stress becomes prolonged and the increased amount of a hormone becomes a destructive agent to your body. Cortisol stimulates appetite by increasing the insulin in your blood stream, which helps maintain your blood sugar. It stimulates the metabolism of fat as well as proteins, and with high levels of stress you keep on gaining weight and it becomes very difficult for you to lose weight. The weight that is gained is more likely to be in the abdominal region; this type of increased weight is associated with a greater risk of heart attacks and strokes.

In a recent study on rainbow trout in Israel, when the fish were exposed to increased cortisol levels, after four to seven days, accelerated aging was found in the cells.

In another study of wild chimpanzees, cortisol was linked to higher rates of male aggressiveness, which makes sense because we know that cortisol is associated with a fight/flight mechanism that all of us have.

One of the early signs of Alzheimer's Disease is damage to the hippocampus region of our brain. The hippocampus region has receptors for cortisol. It is also responsible for our memory.

With increased level of cortisol, we can develop atrophy of the hippocampus that is causing memory impairment. The August 2002 issue of *The Journal of Clinical Endocrinology,* a five-year study was published which linked impaired memory to high levels of cortisol.

You can see from all of the above studies, that increased stress is bad for you and can cause many physical and cognitive changes that are destructive to your body. High levels of stress slowly destroy your body from the inside.

Mental stress can be devastating to your psyche. How do you react to stress? And how do you get rid of that stress? Some people take pills, others engage in dangerous activity, others just try to talk it out, while others go on binge eating sprees and put on weight. Yoga and meditation have been used for a long time for stress reduction and to clear the mind.

If we can reduce that stress by physical activity, we will become much healthier individuals. We will substitute positive energy for negative energy. Our cells will be happy. A happy cell leads to a healthy body.

One of the best activities I have found for stress reduction is dancing. No matter how stressed you are, by the time you finish your dance lesson, or the group dance, you will have forgotten most of what caused you to be stressful.

I once was tremendously stressed. I had patients back to back, all of them had major problems that they had to discuss with me and have resolved.

At the same time, I had many other things to do at home. I felt overloaded. What did I do? I remembered there was a dance party that evening at the local dance club, so I went to it, and over a period of about an hour, danced my stress away. By the time I finished I felt good. When I got home I was able to address the issues I had to complete without being all wound up.

Many people, after working all day, go to happy hour to unwind. They don't care that much about drinking, but it seems to calm them down and prepare them for the rest of the day. Consider my solution the happy *dance* hour. I certainly received many more benefits from that hour of dancing than I would have sitting at some bar drinking alcohol. I was physically active, I had fun, and the stress just melted away from my body.

You know people who constantly worry; the ones who have one problem after another and they always talk about how stressed they are. Why not suggest to those friends of yours to take weekly dance lessons and see what happens to them. You'll probably notice that they stop worrying and start having a lot more fun. You'll see them become happier, better adjusted, and more positive people.

As mentioned earlier, yoga and meditation are great stress reducers. Dancing gives you the same type of mind clearing that you can get from those activities. Listening to the music, moving to the rhythm, improving your balance and muscle tone and joint strength and bone strength, at the same time that you are really having great fun, is the best thing you can do for your body to relieve it from the stresses it is exposed to on a daily basis. Like the song says, "Don't worry, be happy." And I say, "Don't worry, *dance* and be happy."

When you are dancing and listening to the music, moving to the motion of the song, you go into a zone that is happy, carefree, and focused on having pleasure—a zone in which you cannot worry. You're having such a good time dancing that you can't be stressful.

Dancing, by the way, doesn't just reduce stress; dancing can prevent stress. Like the doctor says, "Take two aspirin and call me in the morning." I say, "Go have a dance and call me in the morning."

CHAPTER 12

Dancing as a Sport

Many of you probably don't know that dancing is recognized as a bona fide Olympic sport. Recently at the Millenium Dance Sport Competition in St. Petersburg, Fla., I observed some of the best, most fit athletes I have ever seen. Yes, *athletes*. These are people, from their teens to their eighties. Dance Sport covers all age brackets. There is a level of competition for every one of us.

Did you know that there are all kinds of levels of achievement that one can reach in dancing? It all depends as to how long you have been taking lessons and at what level you have mastered the dance steps. For example, there is the bronze level, the silver level and the gold level. Inside of each one of those levels, there are also sub levels. You start out as a beginner and then you move your way up to the bronze level.

The three days of competitive dancing at the Millenium Dance Competition were divided into various styles of dances. The first day was the **American Smooth Division**, which included dances such as the fox trot and the waltz. The second day the **American Rhythm Division**, which included dances such as the swing and the cha-cha. And the third day was the **International Division.** That division had some of the same dances as the American Division, but also included dance styles such as Paso Double, Viennese waltz, and jive in it. Dancing, when taken outside the social realm and into the sports arena, becomes a highly competitive precise, as well as creative, athletic event. The dance training is as demanding as training for a major athletic event such as a basketball game or tennis match. At the athletic competitive level, the dance style is taken to a level way beyond that of a social dance. A competitive rumba looks totally different from a social rumba. The same is true for the cha-cha or any other social dance.

When I was watching, a series of competitors in the Latin division performed the same dance. Each couple did the dance differently, using their own creative artistic abilities to choreograph the steps to the music. No two couples danced the same way.

During this Dance Sport competition, I made it a point to go every single day and spend a few hours observing the competitors. Every competitor competed against other people at the same level of expertise. For example, bronze level entrants competed against other bronze levels entrants from all around the eastern United States. No matter your level of dancing, you can always join the competitive aspect of dancing and compete with your peer group.

In order for you to become proficient at any level, you have to spend many hours practicing your moves so that you refine every aspect of body movement, coordination and balance that is necessary to make that particular dance look good. At the most competitive levels, such as the international standard dance amateur division, or the international or rhythm Latin division, I saw some of the fittest, thinnest, well-toned bodies ever. These dancers were trim, slim, beautiful, fit, gorgeous, and extremely athletic. The energy they expended to do a fast dance proficiently in the three to four minutes of the dance, caused all of them to pant and perspire profusely. The head, arms, chest, torso, hips and legs are all moving in various directions to get that extra flare to the dance. I can only contrast club and social dancing to competitive dancing as a picnic baseball game to that of a Major League baseball game. Members at the picnic and the stadium all know how to play baseball. Members of both groups play the same positions. The difference is the skill level at which the game is played.

In dancing, you add yet another component to the skill level, that of the artistic-creative component of the dance itself. The professional competitive dancer—the sport dancer—dances from a choreographed routine that is very individual to him and his partner, unlike the social dancer who dances a basic social pattern that everyone can follow to that particular dance.

During the Millenium Dance Sport Competition, I was walking through the hallway near where a number of the competitors were warming up and discussing their workout regimens with one another. I heard all types of discussions: the type of weight lifting routines they went through, the type of nutrition to tone their body so it had no fat, what gave the greatest amount of flexibility so that they could exercise their dance routines most efficiently. It reminded me of listening to bodybuilders talk about the type of proteins they ate and the diets they had in order to build muscle mass so their physiques would look good.

A dancer's biggest concern is being able to stay flexible, well toned, and trim. Think of ballet dancers. They are all thin, and have excellent muscle tone. They take great pride in their appearance and posture. Their bodies are highly tuned to perform at optimum efficiency during the entire ballet. They must appear feather light, as if floating on air, the women graceful, the men strong. They also must maintain poise throughout the entire performance.

Individuals who dance competitively as a sport, have to do the same thing. They have to make the particular dance they are dancing look effortless and beautiful. To do that requires a great amount of skill and self confidence in their abilities to deliver the best show possible for the judges.

Dancing as a sport brings out the competitive spirit and gives you a level of satisfaction after you have mastered a particular dance style. When you take dancing from the social level to the sport level, you move the dance up several notches to where everything has to be done to perfection. From the way your body looks, to the way you carry yourself, to the way your clothes look on you, to the weight lifting gym and nutritional schedule you have to follow, everything ties in to make a sport dancer a finely tuned racing machine.

Like a thoroughbred running the Kentucky Derby, a competitive sport dancer has to perform at maximum peak efficiency to look good, be poised, and exert the tremendous energy required to make a dance look beautiful and effortless. To give you a personal perception of how hard the dance athlete works at his or her sport, try doing 100 sit ups as fast as you can, smiling broadly between each one, at the same time making the sit ups appear effortless. That is exactly what a dance athlete has to do.

Competitive dancing is not for everyone, but for those few of you who really enjoy dancing, it is a means to show off your skills and perfect your abilities. In the end, you will feel good about yourself because of your accomplishments. You can play basketball against your garage with a bunch of friends and have a great time, or you can play basketball in a professional division and have a good time. The only difference is the skill level required. Both of them will give you a tremendous amount of pleasure and it is up to you to decide at what level you want to play.

You do not have to be a professional dancer to have a good time dancing. If you feel you are good at dancing, and you have natural talent, by all means, go ahead and try competing in an event. You'll get a great deal of satisfaction in knowing that you can become really good at something you truly enjoy.

CHAPTER 13

Use It or Lose It

This past week a friend of mine asked if he could use my truck to haul some furniture for reupholstering. I said sure, and didn't think much of it. When I went to start the truck to make sure the battery wasn't dead, I noticed that the right rear tire was flat. As I was taking the wheel off to replace it with the spare, I noticed that the steel belts had peeled off in one area, just like an onion would be peeled.

That's strange, I thought, to have a tire suddenly go flat just sitting there! I hadn't used the truck in months. It's an older Suburban that gets little use during the year, used, as it is, primarily to get things for my house when I have projects, or take the lawn mower or outboard motor in for repair. I couldn't remember when the last time I drove it. This year it just sat most of the time.

After replacing the tire, I thought I'd drive to the tire store to get a new spare to replace the one I had used. During the drive, I noticed my steering wheel was shaking a little bit. That seemed strange; it hadn't done that the last time I drove it. A couple of miles later I became concerned and stopped on the side of the road. Maybe a lug nut was loose on the tire rim of one of the front tires.

The lug nuts were on tight; there was no play in the tires.

On careful inspection of the right front tire, I noticed one area that was smoother than the rest, and the tread appeared to be gone. It reminded me of a small aneurysm trying to come to the surface of the tire.

The tires had adequate tread on them but why was one area slightly raised? I thought to myself, *this is not a good thing!* I'd better take the truck back and take that tire off to get repaired.

At the tire shop the mechanic rolled the tire and noticed the slight bulge.

"The steel belts are going bad," he said, "and the tire's expanding more in one area. I'll get you a new one."

How lucky, I thought, that I found that out. The tire could have blown while I was driving and caused an accident.

I took the tire home and that evening proceeded to put it on my truck late at night. I called my friend and told him I'd be able to help him; that I'd drive the truck over the following day.

On driving to his place, there was still a slight shake to the wheel. It went away at faster speeds. However, to be on the safe side, I drove on side streets rather than the highway.

After we unloaded the furniture he had me haul, I went back to the tire store to see if the wheels needed balancing. They jacked up the truck and right away noticed that the left front tire had a significant bulge at the end of the treads. That's why the steering wheel shook.

I couldn't believe it! Three tires, all bad at the same time. How could this happen? I'd been using the truck about once a month for the past few years, and all of a sudden, all of the tires go bad?

It didn't make sense.

"How long's the truck been sitting outside, unused?" the tire mechanic asked.

"I don't know. Maybe six—seven months."

"You know, with the heat and humidity, and the rain, here in Florida, it's very harsh on rubber. Your rims have started to rust. I could've changed three tires in the time it's taken me to take one of yours off the rim," he complained. "I've had to replace the valve stems, too, 'cause they kept on leaking even after I put the new ones on."

Three of my tires developed aneurysms because the steel belts broke. Why? Because of lack of use.

When a tire sits in one spot, for a long time, with a lot of weight on it, it develops a hollow spot in the tire that weakens the steel belts.

The tread was good because I rarely used the truck, but it was that lack of use for a prolonged time that caused the tires to deteriorate; to get aneurysms through the steel belts.

Does this remind you of anything?

Consider this: We get aneurysms in our blood vessels that can rupture and cause a stroke.

We can die from those aneurysm ruptures just as we can die from a tire blowing up as we are driving.

If I hadn't noticed the problem when I did, one or both of my front tires could have blown and caused a severe accident that might have killed or injured me and others.

The lack of use of my truck caused an essential component breakdown, my tires. Without functioning tires you can't use the truck in a safe manner; without functioning muscles and joints and nerves, you can't walk.

You must constantly use your body to keep it from wearing out. Like I have said over and over, *If you don't use it, you lose it.*

The story doesn't end here.

As I was getting ready to leave the tire store, I asked the owner of the garage to look at my other rear tire (by now, like any normal person, I was getting paranoid).

He looked, and noticed a small crack next to the rim.

"Someone's looking after you," he said. "This tire's ready to blow at any minute."

The crack, a stress crack, went down almost through the entire thickness of the tire, and was ready to pop at any moment. Needless to say, I had him put on a new tire, now the fourth one to be replaced, *because I hadn't used the truck for months.*

How lucky it was that nothing serious happened and that I noticed something wrong, and did something about it, right away. I could have ignored the problem. I could have driven the truck with my steering wheel shaking slightly, thinking it was just a balance problem. I could have driven on the expressway, where the tires would have heated up and blown. Ignoring those early warning signs could have had me and possibly others killed or severely injured in an accident. Someone *was* looking out after me, and wanted me to write the story in this book for others to see.

The garage mechanic told me to use the truck at least once a month, even if it's just to drive to the grocery store, in order to put some use on the tires and keep them from developing weak spots.

Our human body has to be used the same way; you constantly have to keep it moving, as I had talked about in previous chapters, to keep it from falling apart. From your joints to your muscles to your brain, you must constantly use them, or else they will break down causing catastrophic results such as a stroke, a heart attack or a broken bone.

At a recent social function I ran into Frank, an ophthalmologist who used to be one of my neighbors. I asked him how old he was and if he was still practicing full time, because I saw him at grand round conferences at the hospital.

Frank told me that he was 73 and still practicing full time, and that his son had joined him in his ophthalmology practice.

"Have you thought of retiring?" I asked.

"Over the years I've watched my colleagues retire and play golf every day and travel all over the world. Six months to a year later, I started seeing them go to every conference possible because they were getting bored. They'd given up their practices, which was their identity, and just playing golf and traveling wasn't intellectually stimulating enough for them.

"After they went to every medical conference for a couple of years they suddenly stopped going," Frank continued. "I didn't know why. A couple of years may pass and I'd run into them at some social function or at the store.... They suddenly became old men."

"I don't want that to happen to me. *That's* why I'm still practicing."

When Frank was my neighbor six years ago, I used to see him jog with his dog every night. He still takes long walks--several miles every day--with his dog.

Frank knows that if he doesn't use it he will lose it like his doctor colleagues have. They stopped moving and stopped challenging their brains.

A few weeks ago at the yacht club bar I noticed a thin elderly man dance very well with this happy lady. After I had danced several dances, that lively woman came up to us.

"I certainly have enjoyed watching you and your partner dance," she told me.

"Thanks," I responded, pleased with her comment. "I really enjoy dancing."

"My dance partner, Lucian, is a musician and song writer. He's having a CD release party next week at the theater. Why don't you come?"

I went. And enjoyed their jazz performance tremendously. When they introduced the members of the band, I discovered that the drummer and leader of the band, who was also the composer of most of the songs, was 83 years old!

He was also that lively great dancer I'd seen at the Yacht Club the week before. His 73-year-old brother was the saxophone player, and his 59-year-old son, the vocalist.

This CD, composed of instrumental jazz, was Lucian's second, and I made sure I bought one of them at the release party. His first CD of original pop songs, was one of the most popular downloads on the Internet.

I enjoyed both CDs immensely.

This man stayed young by dancing, composing his music and playing his drums on a weekly basis in a band on Sunday nights.

Through the variety of music and lyrics Lucian composed, he kept his mind active and challenged. Through dancing and playing his drums, he kept his body at maximum peak performance, guaranteeing he'd have good reflexes, balance and stamina to enjoy the rest of his life without diseases or physical restrictions.

As you see from these few examples, the worst thing you can do to yourself is to do nothing. You have to use every aspect of your body and if you can't use it then rehabilitate it to where you can use it.

Or you will lose it.

We want to be healthy and we want to be happy. It's a lot easier to be happy if you are healthy.

Health is not a given right; it has to be earned through diligent use of all of our body parts and systems. From the type of foods we eat, as I talk about in the *7 SECRETS OF ANTI-AGING,* to the exercise we do on a regular basis, your quality of life will be directly proportional to the effort you put in now by keeping yourself active and mentally stimulated.

If you don't use your body then you will lose your body. Just like I almost lost my truck and possibly my life, by simply not using it.

CHAPTER 14

Dance for Social Interaction

Social interaction is defined as a dynamic, changing sequence of social actions between individuals or groups of individuals who modify their actions and reactions due to the actions by their interaction partner(s). People attach meaning to a situation, interpret what others mean, and respond accordingly to that situation. Society is organizing to predictable relationships. In other words, patterns in which people respond to each other.

These patterns of behavior establish social order in our society. Some of the expected components of social interaction between others may be respect for others, honesty, a certain degree of tolerance, kindness, and courtesy. Interpersonal relationships rely heavily upon these components. Interacting with others is inbred into the human psyche; from preschool to adulthood, we interact with other human beings. That interaction is an important component of our mental well being.

There is a research journal article of an experiment involving rats, where part of their brain blood supply was cut off. The purpose was to find out how different environments would affect the rate of recovery. The rats that had social interaction and physical activity recovered significantly better <u>in all tests</u> than the group of rats that did not have stimulation through social interaction.

Social interaction is not only important for our psychological well-being, it also is important in improving recovery time after an injury. We need social interaction with others to heal physically as well as psychologically.

We have a need to belong. There is a need within us for interpersonal attachment. We want to belong to a group or organization. Lack of this attachment or belonging or social interaction can have adverse effects on our health, ability to adjust and our well-being.

People need social interaction. We are designed from the ground up to be social animals. We are not designed to be loners, spending all of our time in front of the television set or computer screen, without interacting with other human beings on a physical level. We need to have physical contact, social contact, and even brief emotional contact with other humans.

In today's world of television and computers, many people end up spending a great deal of time alone, being entertained by a screen. They have developed solitary lives that do not involve other humans. It is extremely important for people to be socially involved with other people, not only for their psychological well-being, but also for their over all health, because we are social creatures.

We are designed to be together in groups.

Society has functioned in groups since the beginning of time. Nomads used to travel in groups together, form little villages and play together. One of the most primitive means in which people got together and had fun was through dance. Dance was used as a spiritual uplifting medium. It was part of religious services in Africa, North and South America, in Europe and in the oldest existing society today, the Aborigines in Australia.

Thousands of years ago, people were gathering together and dancing. They were dancing to the Gods, and they were dancing to have fun as a group. Dancing has always been a means by which people could get together and have a wonderful time. The need for social interaction through dance is built into our genes. It is a means of personal expression and it also a means by which the opposite sexes can get together and have good, clean fun.

Dance has been the primary means of social interaction since the beginning of civilization. From the local rec center dance, to the high school dance, to the debutante ball, we still do use dancing as a means to be seen, and to see others. We have used dancing as a means to get together with other people and enjoy each other's company. We have used dancing as a means by which we could actually touch other people of the opposite sex in a non-threatening environment. The ability to be close to another human being of the opposite sex for a few minutes is a safe way in which we can interact with another, yet be able to go away afterwards without any repercussions.

Through dancing, we can have fun with a total stranger, and when the dance is done, we can go back to our group of friends knowing that we do not have to be involved with that stranger any more, even though we had a wonderful time with that person for that brief period of time.

We need to have an excuse to go out and shop for a beautiful dress or suit, to buy beautiful jewelry, makeup, perfume, and all of the things needed to make us look the best possible. Going to a dance gives us that excuse.

People go to dances looking good. When you look good, you feel good. You feel good about yourself because you feel good about your appearance, and you feel good because you know you are going to have a good time dancing. How many people do you know who met at a dance, where the first words that they spoke to each other were, "May I have this dance?" Your parents may have even met that way, and that's why you exist. They met that way because they went dancing.

From ancient civilizations to modern society, dancing has been the primary means for us humans to get together and socialize. Dancing has been the primary means for us to meet the opposite sex and form bonds, some of which became lasting and ended up in lifetime relationships.

In today's society, many people are living alone. They get into the rut of the same routine every day, watching the same television programs, and going about their daily chores. It is not good for man—or woman—to be alone.

If you go dancing, you don't have to be alone.

Many ballrooms and dance studios throw social parties on a regular basis.

The social interaction that you get from dancing is vital to your existence. It gives you something to look forward to. It allows you to go out and have fun and interact with people who also want to have fun. Between dances you end up talking to people sitting next to you and you find out about their lives. You may also have snacks and refreshments, but most of all, you will enjoy yourself by either dancing, or watching other people dance. If you see moves that you think you would like to learn, you will sign up for more dance lessons so that you can become proficient at them. The process of signing up for more dance lessons, or taking another group class, allows you to get out further and be more involved with other people. It is a snowball effect. One dance leads to another, and that dance leads to yet another, and before you know it you have become a proficient dancer.

Not only that, but dancing helps get rid of boredom. Dancing gives you an excuse to get out. It gives you an excuse to get away from a boring existence. It gives you an excuse to dress up and look good and it allows you to meet other people and interact with them in a pleasant environment.

You'll find that people who dance, are generally very nice. They are pleasant, courteous, and are fun to be around. You almost never meet grumpy people at a dance. The dancers you meet are fun loving and active. Those you meet at a dance party are people who want to have a good time, people who want to exercise and people who like being with other people. Like the song goes, people who need other people are the luckiest people in the world. We need other people in our lives to be happy. Dancing allows you to meet other people through which you have something in common with, which is dancing. These people are fun loving people, outgoing people, and people who are active. These people take care of themselves, they watch what they eat, and they are concerned about their appearance. Dancers love to have fun, love to laugh, and love to move to the music. Don't you want to be around people like that? I certainly do. When I am around fun loving people who are dancing, I feel good. All of my troubles disappear and I become surrounded by the positive dancing environment.

Many widows benefit greatly by going out and dancing. Going to dance parties gets them out of the house, gives them exercise, and allows them to develop family type bonds between other dancers. Their loneliness disappears because they have something to look forward to, the Tuesday night dance or the Friday night dance, or the Saturday afternoon social.

Dancing un-clutters the cobwebs in your brain, causes your brain and muscles to grow, strengthens your bones and strengthens your psyche by allowing you to be socially involved with other people.

Dancing is a win-win situation.

The other night I went to one of the older studios in the area that had primarily an older crowd. I talked with women in their 70's and 80's, all of whom were very active and good dancers and I was amazed at how beautifully dressed all of these older ladies and gentlemen were. The pride that they took in themselves to have the perfect hairdo, the beautiful dress and the stylish shoes and accessories was astounding. When I asked these ladies to dance, their faces lit up. They were eager to go on the dance floor and float to the music. As we danced, I saw them become young people again. Their spirits rose, and smiles came upon their faces. They loved dancing with a partner. They loved being on the dance floor and they loved moving to the music.

Dance parties from dance studios, dance halls or ballrooms, will usually have at least two or three mixers during the evening, where the ladies line up on one side of the room and the gentlemen on the other. One by one the gentlemen take whichever lady comes next in line and dances once around the ballroom with her. The mixer allows all the people in the hall to dance. Generally there are more ladies than gentlemen, so the men end up dancing twice as much as the women. It is a non-selective process, and whoever comes up next in line is the person you dance with. They may be a good dancer, they may be a mediocre to poor dancer, but you dance with them anyway because that is dance etiquette. A mixer allows people to get out and dance randomly with whomever is available.

A steal dance does the same thing. The music stops and you have to find a new partner on the dance floor. If you are sitting down when the music stops, you go to the dance floor and ask one of the other partners away (steal them) from whomever they are dancing with. Both mixers and steal dances allow you to dance with a large variety of partners without waiting to have someone ask you, or you having to go out and ask someone to dance. You just get out there, stay in the line and take the next person in line and dance with them. It's as simple as that.

You don't have to be a good dancer to do this because in about three minutes or so you'll be finished dancing with that person, and you can go on to the next.

Mixers allow social interaction between total strangers in a very safe, non-threatening environment.

That touch of another human being is very important to us. It is healing, it is soothing, and it is calming. We need to be touched by other humans. Dancing allows us to get out and be touched and also to touch others and interact with them. We all need social interaction.

I cannot think of any better way to get out and interact with a large group of people than by going dancing. Whatever kind of dancing you prefer, just getting out there and dancing with others will allow you to maintain contact with other humans. That human contact is so important for psychological and physical well being. A baby needs human touch to grow and thrive. When we get older, we need human touch to keep us alive and to thrive. By dancing, we touch someone and they touch us while we glide to the music and enjoy ourselves in unison.

CHAPTER 15

Dancing for Relationship Enhancement and Romance

People who have been married a long time get into routines and start taking each other for granted. Many couples become stressed out and very tense because of financial problems, family problems, and job problems. These tensions can eventually erode a loving relationship and make it dull, predictable and boring. When people become so engrossed in their responsibilities of just living, they start to ignore each other as a couple. They take each other for granted and their partner becomes just another equation in their existence. Their partner becomes someone that is expected to do a certain number of things around the house or at their job, or at their church, or with their kids, or with fixing things, or with being a provider. Their partner no longer is a source of joy, pleasure, excitement and romance in their life. Their partner just becomes a bread earner, or a homemaker, or someone to do things with so that you don't have to be alone. Romance has disappeared.

How would you define romance? Everyone has their own definition or their own concept of what is romantic. That concept is based upon what they see in the movies or on television, and it is also based upon their perception of someone's gestures. It is the little things that are romantic to the receiver.

A woman may find a gentleman opening her door for her as being romantic. Those tiny little cards with love notes on them, or the small little bouquets left at her night stand before leaving for work. These little gestures mean *I am thinking of you, I care about you, and I want you to be special in my life.*

What makes candlelight dinners so romantic? It isn't the candle and it isn't the dinner. It is the mood that is created between two people, where they can connect. That special mood is perceived as romance. It is a time where two people can focus on each other 100%. It is a setting. It facilitates the interaction between the couple, where their hormones perk up and they start feeling very loving toward one another. Dancing and music sets up the same environment. It is very hard to think of anything else other than the music and the dance when you are dancing with your partner. You look at your partner, you hold them, and you start moving in unison to a pattern that makes the dance look good. The pattern may be a waltz, a rumba, or a tango.

The romantic component of dancing lies in the beauty of two people interacting and moving together as a unit. The beauty of two people touching each other, looking at each other, gliding in unison and enjoying each other's company for the duration of the dance.

When you finish dancing you feel good, your partner feels good, and you both had a wonderful time because you clicked. You clicked at a level that fulfilled your basic human need of connection. It is a gut reaction to the dance and the music, and the movement itself. It has existed since the beginning of time. Dancing lifts your spirits and elevates your mood, *and you are sharing that feeling with someone else.* This sharing of the movement, the music, the touching, the gliding, the sensuality, creates romance. The romance may be short lived, lasting the duration of the dance, or it may enhance an existing relationship that is budding into a beautiful flower.

Dancing is the process of the opening of each rose petal, one at a time, until the entire beauty of the flower is revealed.

Did you know that more women prefer a night of dancing to receiving flowers or chocolates on Valentine's Day? Most men would consider sending their special lady flowers on special occasions. Very few would consider taking them dancing. However, dancing, to women, is as romantic as any gesture you can do to show your affection.

Dancing can rekindle stressed out, worn out relationships, where everything is mundane. It adds a spark to the relationship. It allows the couple to connect again on a physical level and on a romantic level, where they both enjoy themselves, moving in unison, touching, laughing, looking at each other, and being happy.

The very act of holding each other, touching, and moving to the music in unison, is a romantic act.

Most people who watch good dancers on a dance floor will immediately notice the romantic component of dance. Women will stare at the dancers and swoon at the beauty of a couple gliding over the dance floor. I remember a dance instructor telling me once that on a scale of 0 to 10, a man will immediately start out at a level of 5 before he says the first word to the lady, if she had watched him dance and he is a good dancer. There is a romantic perception how the well polished man dances, and an experienced lady dances. Dancing is considered a beautiful act, an act where two humans move in unison, gracefully gliding on the dance floor, just like Cinderella glided with her prince at his castle.

I have seen many couples on the dance floor who light up when they start dancing. When the evening is finished, they are both happy and content with one another. They have enjoyed an experience that cannot be described in words. They have mutually participated in an event that created joy in their inner being. Any stresses they had prior to going dancing were relieved after they danced together for a while. They refocused on themselves as a couple, and put all of their worries behind them.

Most problems we have in our lives are non-significant, little irritations that clog up our mind with worry. They add stress to our lives. They prevent us from truly enjoying each other as a couple.

When a couple gets on the dance floor, it is a freeing environment. All of the problems are left behind them and the only thing that is in front of them is the music, the dance floor, and the motion they create as they glide together in unison. It is like going into a trance that is pleasant, enjoyable, and romantic.

Several years ago, I was at a Christmas party sitting next to a lady I'd often seen walking in the mornings for exercise. She was in her early 90's and very much mentally alert and physically fit. I would pass by her in the mornings and she would smile and say *Good morning,* but I never had the opportunity to engage her in a conversation. During this Christmas party, we started talking about a variety of things and eventually the topic came to her late husband.

She fairly glowed as she told me how wonderful a man he was. Although he had been dead a number of years, she still talked about him with raving enthusiasm.

"What made your relationship with this man so wonderful?" I asked.

"He was such a fine man," she answered. "He was so romantic. When we were watching a television program where a song was sung or an orchestra was playing, he would take me off the sofa and start dancing with me. It was so romantic. He just swept me off my feet."

The very act of her husband asking her to dance on her living room floor was perceived by her as being one of the most romantic gestures he could do. They connected, held each other, and enjoyed touching as they danced back and forth to the music in their own living room. Twenty years after he died, she still remembered those little romantic dance gestures. The remembrance made her feel good. It made her feel happy. It made her feel desirable, and it made her feel romantic toward her husband.

In our hectic, stressed out, multi-tasking world, few of us slow down to smell the roses. We run from one activity to the next, from one chore to the next, one responsibility to another. Rarely do we just slow down and enjoy each other as a couple. By stopping what you are doing, taking your partner in your hands and dancing a beautiful dance to music that you both enjoy, you rekindle the romance. You start appreciating each other more because you are doing *Something Special Together*.

Everything else is put aside. The only thing that counts is you and your partner. You move together as a unit. You forget all of your worries because you are dancing. You feel connected with your partner again. The woman feels appreciated and the man feels wanted.

Men want to please the special lady in their lives and women want to feel like they are special to their man. They want to feel that they are appreciated, cared for and loved.

One of the best ways that a man can show that feeling is by asking his lover to dance. By holding her in his arms, she will feel secure; she will feel special; she will feel happy and a romantic feeling will start to blossom.

Recently I went to a business luncheon with a doctor who had been married seven years, who told me that his wife, a dentist, had been wanting to learn to dance with him for a long time. She watches every dance show on television because she loves to watch the people move to the music, and the beauty of the dance. She finds dancing romantic and very enjoyable.

He said they'd discussed learning to dance two years before they were married. That was nine years ago and they still hadn't taken dance lessons! His ears perked up when I told him that dancing was one of my hobbies, and my primary means of exercise. We ended up spending the rest of our business lunch discussing dancing, dance studios, and dance styles. He was excited because he knew nothing about the dance world. He didn't know you could take group lessons and learn to dance relatively inexpensively. He didn't know there were dance packages available to take private lessons and group lessons, and enjoy dance parties with other like-minded individuals.

When our luncheon ended, I gave him a brochure I happened to have from a dance studio I'd attended.

"My wife is going to be happy because after all this time I am going to do something with her she's wanted to do since we first met."

Many women love to dance. They want their partner to dance with them, and they are so happy when their partner, a boyfriend or husband, takes an interest in what they like to do. No matter how stressed out your life may be, how complicated your home situation is, cares disappear when you get on the dance floor and start dancing. You can be unhappy, you can be stressed, you can be worried, but when you dance, you forget everything. You are put into another mood. A mood that is happy, a mood that is romantic, a mood that makes you feel like there are no worries, there are no problems, and you can relax and enjoy each other.

Several months ago, I called my good friend, Harold, whom I hadn't seen for a couple of years. He had retired and moved to a retirement community in Sun City, Fla.

"What have you been doing," I asked, "still sailing, playing tennis?"

"You wouldn't believe what I'm doing. I took up dancing and it is one of the best things I have ever done."

He raved about the dance classes he takes with his wife, the parties they go to, the dance instructors, and the fun he and his wife and other couples are having. He couldn't stop talking about the dancing that they were doing together, and how much excitement it had added to their lives and their relationship. Now they had someplace to go and an activity to participate in where they both had a good time.

Dancing rekindled their relationship after many years of marriage. They met new friends through dancing, and their social world opened up to new experiences that they never knew existed.

Dancing is an excellent way to rekindle the romance and enhance your relationship. It is an excellent way to develop a romantic relationship. It is an excellent way to start to enjoy life again.

CHAPTER 16

Dance for Self Preservation - Taking Care of Yourself

What does *self-preservation* mean? Let's get back to the basics.

What do we do when we preserve something? What are preserves?

Well, if you eat breakfast every morning, you may have strawberry *preserves* or jam on your toast.

The normal thing that happens to strawberries once they turn ripe is oxidation, which turns to spoilage. Spoilage turns to mold, the mold eats up the strawberry, small little critters come by and eat the mold and the remainder of the strawberry, and before you know it, the bacteria have eaten up the whole strawberry.

Sometimes a worm comes along and feasts of that strawberry, too.

However, if you put that strawberry in some kind of solution with sugar and cook it, and add a few key ingredients, that strawberry will be preserved for a long time in a jar.

It will still be red and it will still taste like a strawberry.

What do we do to preserve a valuable painting? We frame it. We tape paper over the back of the frame so bugs can't get behind the painting and eat it up. We keep it in an air-conditioned, humidity-controlled room. We keep it out of the sunlight. And, occasionally, we touch it up when it starts to fade or crack.

Self-preservation goes back in various societies for thousands of years. The wealthy Egyptians spent a great deal of money preserving their bodies for the afterlife. Ancient South American Indians embalmed bodies as well, wrapping them in oils and cloths, so that they would be in good shape for the afterlife.

One of the most well preserved human bodies I have ever seen was in Moscow.

Lenin's tomb is underground in a glass-covered vault in Red Square. All the oxygen was removed from the vault so there was nothing to destroy his flesh, and he looked as he must have when he was alive, over 75 years ago. A team of scientists are in charge, making sure that Lenin's body will remain in its original state for viewing by generations to come.

Lenin's hair was perfect and so were his eyelashes, his mouth and his skin. Even the stubble in his chin, where hair used to grow, was visible. He is perfectly preserved.

However, what good does it do us to preserve our dead bodies since we won't be able to enjoy them.

What we do want, is to preserve our *present* bodies in their live state, so that we can get maximum benefit out of them. Now. You deserve it. You have worked all your life to save up for retirement. You don't want to spend all of your hard earned savings on doctor visits, nursing homes, nursing assistance, wheelchairs and walkers, do you?

I certainly don't.

So, what are you going to do about it. Since you're reading this book, you are certainly not one of those couch potatoes who sits around all day watching television, are you? You are most likely an active person who wants to enjoy life as much as possible. You want to live life to its fullest. You want to stay active and enjoy yourself for as long as it is physically and mentally possible.

In order for you to extend your active life and have as much fun as you possibly can, you have to preserve your body. You have to preserve your mind and you have to preserve your spirit.

We want to preserve our core being for as long as possible. This does not mean that we can't do an occasional touchup here and there, either through cosmetic procedures, or through esthetic applications of various creams and make-ups, but none of these procedures will do you any good unless your core is intact.

Think of a car. You can give it a paint job, new tires, new chrome, new upholstery, new windshield wipers and new exhaust tailpipe, but none of these external additions are going to do your car any good unless the engine, transmission, and the drive shaft and differentials work. The core has to work before anything else works

The same thing goes with your body. You have to function as a biological being. Your digestive system has to work. That means you have to be able to take the food in, digest it properly, and excrete it properly. Your circulatory system has to work. That means your blood has to flow through all the vessels without being clogged somewhere by obstructions, and your ticker, your heart, has to work efficiently to pump all the blood through the miles and miles of blood vessels. You need to feed all your cells in your body. Your lungs have to work. Without your lungs, the blood can't get any oxygen, which your cells need for survival.

Your blood takes the oxygen from the lungs and the nutrients from your intestinal system and feeds your cells so they can live. Without food to your cells, the cells will starve and die. When the cells die, you die. It is a very basic system in principle. However, the implementation of our biological bodies to work efficiently, is very complicated.

There are billions of cells in your body that have to work effectively in order for you to survive and be healthy. Your body is going through constant transitions.

Did you know that every month you have all new skin cells? Every month you are reborn on the outside.

Did you know that every three months you have all new bone cells? Your skeleton becomes a new skeleton every three months.

We are constantly growing new cells and eliminating old cells. If you say to yourself, I'm too old to do this, well, in three months you will be another person. Biologically, that is.

You are never too old to change.

Your body is constantly changing, and what you put into it and how you treat it, will be displayed in how you feel and how you look from thirty days to ninety days from now. We are constantly going through changes in our bodies. How the new cells grow, how healthy they are, and how well they function, is entirely dependent upon how we treat our body.

You've heard the saying in connection with computers, "garbage in equals garbage out." So, too, for our bodies. Not only do our bodies need proper nutrition and healthy nutrition, to survive and prosper; our bodies need proper stimulation through exercise in order to train those new body parts to be efficient and healthy.

Let's go into the practical aspect of what we need for self preservation on an every day level. To survive, we need air, food, and water. At this level, we can be sustained in a hospital bed with tubes tied to our body, and a respirator pumping us air. If we want to go above this level, which all of us do, we need to add mental acuity and mobility to this equation.

Without that mental acuity, we can't enjoy the mobility. Without the mobility, we can't enjoy the mental acuity.

In other words, you have to be aware of your surroundings, and you have to be able to enjoy your surroundings.

Just because you are aware of your surroundings does not necessarily mean that you can fully enjoy them. You need to be mobile and be able to do things to fully enjoy your environment. *Physical activity is a key ingredient for prolongation of life.* This is where dancing comes into play.

Dancing stimulates your mind in many ways.

It forces you to become mentally sharp. It is extremely difficult to learn and retain the patterns that you learn in various dances. It takes a long time. It takes concentration. What makes it enjoyable is listening to the music and getting a spiritual uplift through combining movement to the music. The repetitive combination of movement and the ethereal aspect of the music gives you a spiritual, uplifting, and mood elevation, and at the same time, mental stimulation. Your mind becomes sharper and more aware of your environment. You are able to think clearer. I have mentioned in previous chapters, dancing is one of the few activities that stimulates mind growth. The other major component is that it stimulates muscle growth, balance, and coordination. It stimulates bone growth and strengthening. It helps prevent falls, and it gives you independence. Your reflexes become sharper. Your mind becomes more acute, and your muscles become stronger and more toned. This combination gives you the freedom of mobility.

Dancing is one of the best physical activities you can engage in to prolong life. Not only do you get the muscle strengthening and bone strengthening benefit of dancing, you also get the psychological benefits of dancing, and mind stimulation benefits of dancing. Through dancing, you not only strengthen your body, you also strengthen your mind. An added bonus to dancing is that you strengthen your psychological well being, because you feel so good when you dance, and you feel so good when you finish dancing, and you feel so good when you drive home and go to bed that night.

Dancing is a great stress reducer. All the things that you thought were bothersome disappear carried away by the music. Your troubles disappear and you focus on what is important in life, which is your family, friends, and your spiritual and psychological well being. Dancing is spiritual, it is uplifting, it has been used in religious services since the beginning of time. And, dancing elevates your mood, so that you become happy. No matter how stressed you are, and how many worries you have, dancing takes them away.

Self-preservation involves psychological preservation, physical preservation, mental preservation, mobility preservation, and overall well-being enhancement.

Dance on a regular basis, and you will actually look better. There will be more circulation to the small capillaries in your face, and you'll develop a glow, which makes you more beautiful. Your lungs will work better, your mind will work better, your coordination will improve, your bone strength will improve, and your muscles and reflexes will be greatly enhanced. Through dancing, you'll be preserving yourself and enhancing your ability to enjoy life.

Life without mobility is a bummer. Life with mobility and freedom of movement and freedom of thought, is a great pleasure. You need to dance to preserve yourself. You need to dance to stay healthy, be alert, and psychologically well balanced. Remember that song, *If You're Happy And You Know It, Clap Your Hands?* Well . . .

If you're happy and you know it, stomp your feet
If you're happy and you know it, clap your hands

If you're happy and you know it
Then your face will surely show it
If you're happy and you know it, then you'll dance!

CHAPTER 17

Dance to Live

What does "to live," mean? For me it means passion. That spark and life that stimulates us to go on and achieve new goals, new pleasures and joys. It means to spark new desires yet to be fulfilled. It is an intense burning to achieve something or do something that you find infinitely rewarding. And note, there's a big difference between "existing" and truly "living."

To live means reaching beyond the ordinary, beyond just mere existence.

Passion is the desire to have fulfillment and continued interest and enjoyment in what you do. Living in itself is primarily existence, i.e., the need of food, shelter, clothing, daily routines that go on day by day until we die. Living for me means experiencing life to its fullest, being mentally and physically active and interested in so many things that there are not enough minutes in the day for you to accomplish everything you want to do each day.

To live means being excited about life, living a life of joy, and being happy, extremely happy.

To live means making the most of every day and making each day as fulfilling and as enjoyable as possible.

We were not meant to live on this earth to be miserable. We were meant to enjoy the fruits of our labor until we breathe our last breath. We were meant to be engaged in life, to be engaged in what we do, to love what we do and always look forward to new things and new horizons, never losing that spark, that interest that makes us fulfilled and satisfied that we are, indeed, *living*.

I believe, and hope I have convinced you, that dancing is one of the best ways of truly living.

The most potent emotion in the universe is love. The more you can be in the state of love, the happier and healthier you will be. Dancing will bring out the joy and love in you. It will make you happy.

If you are in love with the person you are dancing with, your love will become stronger, and your enjoyment of each other will reach levels of ecstasy that you never imagined. You will live in a state far more fulfilling than 99% of the people on this earth.

If your partner is not a lover, but a friend, or even an acquaintance met at the dance, you will still enjoy the benefits of dancing together, of touching one another, of gliding across the floor in step to the music.

Dance lessens the distance between individuals.

By dancing, you will be physically active and mentally active, because you will be constantly learning new steps. The physical activity through dance will burn calories, strengthen your bones, strengthen your muscles, improve your coordination, improve your balance, strengthen your ligaments, and cause your mind to grow.

In order to live fully, you have to have a capability to enjoy life. In order to have that capability, you need to have the physical ability to have mobility to be able to go out and do things, to have the stamina to stay up late and dance, or enjoy an evening with friends at a ball game or a soccer match, or carousing about town.

You have to have the physical stamina to travel the world and explore new places, visit other cultures, be engaged in activities you have always wanted to do throughout your life, but you never have the time to do. Dancing will improve your health enormously, and allow you to do the things you have always dreamed of doing. Dancing will allow you to make new friends, be involved, and get a life. If you are living by yourself and have nowhere to go, find the closest dance studio near you, a studio that offers regular parties where you can interact with other people who enjoy dancing. Dancing will get you out of the house. Dancing will stimulate you to be more interested in living. You will look forward to the nights that you get to dress up and go to a dance party. You will look forward to a beautiful sunset. You will look forward to the next activity that you want to do. You will be excited about enjoying your retirement, excited about spending a beautiful evening with your partner, dancing the night away and being totally lost in the music, the rhythms, and the touch and feel of your partner. Dancing brings out the endorphins, the happy hormones within you. You will feel good mentally and physically. You will have increased energy because your body will be conditioned to do many more things in life than you ever dreamed were possible. You will have a positive mental attitude. You will get rid of that "stinking thinking," and replace it with positive thoughts that will allow you to enjoy your life to its fullest.

No matter what you are doing—volunteer work, working a full time job, or a part time job—dancing will allow you to function better at whatever you are doing, because it will relieve any stresses that you have, and allow you to start fresh each day, looking forward to whatever happens that day. If you don't believe me, try it.

Pick the most stressful day that you have; at the end of it, go to a dance party or take a group dance lesson and see how you feel at the end of that lesson. Your stresses will just melt away. For example, I remember having a tremendously stressful day. I went into my office and there was a letter sitting on my desk. It was a resignation from one of my key employees who had been with me for ten years. At the same time, I had to pay a couple of very expensive insurance bills, which had greatly increased because of the hurricanes that we recently had in Florida. But that wasn't all. Every one of my patients had tremendous problems of their own. Their lives were falling apart; they were in severe pain; they weren't able to work, and they were all stressed out because of their personal problems that they related to me. When the day was over, my shoulders were heavy. Not only did I have my own unexpected problems to deal with, I had dealt with everyone else's problems at the same time. I had to worry about finding a replacement for my staff worker in a very short period of time, placing ads, interviewing new people, wondering if they were going to work out or not, how was the other staff going to react to them, and so on. It was a very stressful time.

That evening I went to the local dance studio to take a private and a group lesson. By the time my lessons were over, I had totally forgotten all of my worries, and they suddenly became insignificant. I was just happy to be enjoying myself, happy to be moving. My head was clear, and I was ready to start the next day with a clean slate.

Dancing provided me with physical exercise and soothed my mental state. Before long, I was concentrating on my partner and the dance, and the calming effect of the music put me at ease, so that I forgot all the stressful problems I had. Dancing allowed me to live. It allowed me to enjoy the rest of the evening with my partner. It took the stress away, and it provided me with physical activity so that my body stayed strong and healthy.

After you have been dancing for a while, not only will you dance to live, but you will live to dance. You will look forward to the times you can go to the dance studio or to a dance function and enjoy yourself. You will look forward to that special time that you can dress up and make yourself all pretty and smell good so that you will look good to your partner, or if you don't have a partner, you will be able to attract other partners to dance with you at the dance party. No matter where you travel in this world, if you look in the local paper, phonebook, or the Internet, and find a dance studio nearby that has functions, your life will be greatly enriched by going to those functions. You will have a community with whom you can do things with, even in a strange place. A place that you had never been to before, but you will suddenly be transformed into being one of them, just by dancing with them. Dancing allows you to live, no matter where you are. It allows you to reach out beyond the ordinary, and to experience music and physical activity with other like-minded individuals, no matter where you are in this world. Dancing allows you to interact with total strangers in a safe environment. It allows you to touch other people. Touch is so healing for our psyche. Dancing allows you to enjoy the moment with people you have never met before. Dancing allows you to be happy with your loved one, or with the partner that you are dancing with. You know you are living when your mind is sharp, your body is physically fit, your energy level is up, and when you have a passion for living.

Once you start dancing on a regular basis, you won't care what is on television. Being able to get out and exercise and have fun at the same time, listening to the music and engaging your dance partner in the dance moves, will take priority over any television program. You will know that what you are doing is healthy for your body, healthy for your mind, and healthy for your spirit. You will have a life, a life that will enhance your memory, improve your balance and coordination, strengthen your bones and muscles, and make your outlook on life positive and exciting.

As you can see from the previous chapters, there are many health benefits to dancing. There are many psychological benefits to dancing. There are many spiritual benefits to dancing, as well. People have used the dance to express joy since the beginning of time, and people continue to use dancing to put them into a happy mental, stress free state, that has benefits that not only lift your spirits, but also lift your body's capacity to function way beyond expectations, in harmony with nature, to a very, very old age.

One time a woman I was dancing with told me how she got into dancing.

"My kids said, 'Mom, you need to get out there and get a life.'"

She'd been staying at home, going out to shop when necessary, and except for watching television, had nothing in particular to do in the evenings. When she discovered dancing, her life was transformed. She became a new person. She became excited about life. She started going to a dance studio on a regular basis, just to have that uplifting high that you get when you dance with others. She suddenly 'had a life,' was involved in an activity that made her happy, an activity that gave her joy and excitement, an activity that will greatly prolong her life.

A while ago, I went to a variety of different dance studios in our region to see how they varied from each other. Each studio develops its own particular style and attracts different groups of people, based upon that style. Some studios have predominantly older people, people who were in their 70's and 80' and 90's and others had middle-aged and younger people. Some studios taught only the American dance style; others taught the International dance style, and some studios taught a variety of both. There are studios for hip-hop music, studios for tap, and a large variety of studios for ballroom dancing, as well as specialized studios for latin dancing or swing dancing. The common denominator that I noticed about all the studios, was how happy and excited the people were when they danced. In some of the studios, the women were anxiously waiting for a gentleman to ask them to dance. When they were asked to dance, they immediately smiled and lit up. It was like a baby receiving a lollipop. That is how dancing immediately transformed the psychological well being. At the swing dances, I noticed the women were constantly asking men to dance, and vice versa. So, no one was sitting around, and everyone was happy dancing to the music. There is no rule that says that only men have to ask ladies to dance. In today's world, women routinely ask men to dance. The women are there just to dance, and so are the men. It is a very safe environment for people to mutually enjoy each other without becoming personally involved. These people have learned that dancing transforms their lives into another dimension. It allows them to live. They are not just merely existing. They are having fun, and improving their health at the same time. They are uplifting their spirits and going home in a peaceful, happy state, where they can get a good night's sleep. They are going home, knowing that what they did was healthy for them and very, very enjoyable for them. Stress reduction is a very important component in anti-aging. Dancing greatly reduces your stress level. By reducing your stress level, you are able to live and enjoy life to it's fullest. When you leave the dance floor, you leave the dance floor with a good mental attitude. You leave the dance floor with a smile.

I think that dancing is an important component in staying young mentally and physically. When you dance you have a win-win situation. You get the tremendous benefit of physical activity in anti-aging as well as well as the psychological, social and spiritual uplifting effects of music. This combined effect is a powerful force for longevity of body, mind and spirit.

I remember a quotation from Margery Curtz, a 98 year-old woman who lived in Naples and danced regularly. "Smile awhile, and while you smile another smiles. And soon, there are miles and miles of smiles, and life is worthwhile because you smiled."

If you are young, I want you to get as much joy out of life as possible by dancing on a regular basis. If you are approaching retirement age, or are in retirement, I want all of you to be like my healthy elderly patients, active, fun loving, alert, and having the best time in life ever.

The End

For further information on longevity please visit   - www.antiagingrevolution.com

7 Secrets of Anti-Aging can be obtained at the above web site and at Amazon.com. The next edition will be called *Seven Secrets of Anti-Aging.*